*"This is something you live with your whole life.
Asthma's part of who I am,
and I can't control it if I don't know about it."*

—CATHI B.

Chicken Soup for the Soul®
Healthy Living:
Asthma

Chicken Soup for the Soul®
Healthy Living:
Asthma

Jack Canfield
Mark Victor Hansen
Norman H. Edelman, M.D.

Health Communications, Inc.
Deerfield Beach, Florida

www.hcibooks.com
www.chickensoup.com

Library of Congress Cataloging-in-Publication Data
available from the Library of Congress

Publisher: Health Communications, Inc.
            3201 S.W. 15th Street
            Deerfield Beach, FL 33442-8190

Cover design by Larissa Hise Henoch
Inside book design by Lawna Patterson Oldfield
Inside book formatting by Dawn Von Strolley Grove

Contents

Fear less, hope more,

eat less, chew more,

whine less, breathe more,

talk less, say more,

love more,

and all good things

will be yours.

—Swedish Proverb

Introduction:
Breathe Easier with Asthma

Today, it seems as though asthma is everywhere. In fact, an estimated 20 million people—6.1 million of them children under 18—currently have asthma. If you are reading this book, then you know someone who suffers from this chronic disease. It could be you, a family member, a young child, a coworker, or a neighbor.

Asthma isn't always obvious; you can't tell an asthma sufferer from looking at them—unless they are having trouble breathing. Though you can't always see asthma, you can see and count its devastating effects. Asthma is the leading serious chronic illness among children. It is the number one cause of school absences attributed to chronic illnesses and accounts for a total of 14 million lost school days each year.

In every community, children and adults suffer from asthma, but in our inner cities, asthma is especially prevalent. In addition, although more prescriptions for asthma medications are being written, many people are not using their medications as prescribed. The result: an increase in asthma attacks that land people in the emergency room.

But the good news is that asthma in most cases *can* be controlled. Every person with asthma can and should expect to lead a normal life. Far too many people with asthma accept limitations on their life. Children accept the fact that they can't participate in gym class. Teenagers accept the fact that they can't do sports. Adults accept the fact that they have to get up twice a night almost every night, gasping for breath.

I want to reach people to make them understand that they should feel better and they can feel better. It's not okay to accept limitations on your life because of asthma. If asthma is holding you back, tell your doctor. Maybe your doctor can change your medication. Maybe you need to use an asthma inhaler before you exercise. Maybe you can make changes at home to get rid of asthma triggers.

One day, perhaps soon, we will be able not only to control asthma but to cure it. Today, there is great reason to hope for a cure for asthma. We have learned so much about asthma in recent years, particularly about the inflammation in the airways that leads to asthma. We have great reason to hope that we can eventually find the key to shutting off this inflammatory process and curing this disease.

But in the meantime, there are many things you

and your doctor can do to control your asthma so you can lead a healthy, normal life. On the following pages you'll learn many ways to control your asthma, like getting rid of asthma triggers in your home, having a plan that will tell you what to do in case you feel an asthma attack coming on, dealing with your child's asthma at home and at school, exercising with asthma, traveling with asthma, plus sections on asthma during the teen years, pregnancy and senior years.

I hope that you will come away from reading this book with tips that will help you or your loved one with asthma to breathe easier. The most important message I can give you about asthma is: you can control it—don't let it control you!

—Norman H. Edelman, M.D.
Chief Medical Officer
American Lung Association

Don't Let Asthma Control You!

Asthma. It means many things to many people. For some, asthma means wheezing during spring allergy season. For others, it means a daily struggle to breathe normally. Asthma affects people differently—some people have mild asthma, some severe.

But it's important for everyone with asthma and their families to know that you can control asthma—don't let it control you! If you're not breathing normally, don't accept it—it's not okay. This book will walk you through the steps you can take to begin to breathe normally again, in many situations, throughout your life.

Yes, most cases of asthma can be controlled. But unfortunately, many people with asthma continue to struggle with their breathing. Perhaps their asthma is being ignored in the hopes that it will simply go away. Or they aren't taking the right kind of medication. Or they aren't taking their medication as often as they should. Maybe they've been told—wrongly—that most people grow out of their asthma.

There are many reasons why people with asthma aren't breathing normally and aren't living life to the fullest. You don't have to be one of those people. You can—and should—live a normal, healthy life despite your asthma.

In fact, several Olympic medalists have had

asthma, including track and field star Jackie Joyner-Kersee and swimmer Tom Dolan. They are proof that asthma doesn't have to slow you down.

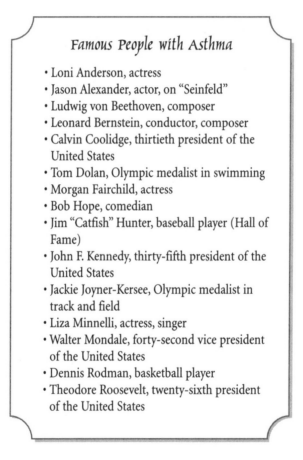

Famous People with Asthma

- Loni Anderson, actress
- Jason Alexander, actor, on "Seinfeld"
- Ludwig von Beethoven, composer
- Leonard Bernstein, conductor, composer
- Calvin Coolidge, thirtieth president of the United States
- Tom Dolan, Olympic medalist in swimming
- Morgan Fairchild, actress
- Bob Hope, comedian
- Jim "Catfish" Hunter, baseball player (Hall of Fame)
- John F. Kennedy, thirty-fifth president of the United States
- Jackie Joyner-Kersee, Olympic medalist in track and field
- Liza Minnelli, actress, singer
- Walter Mondale, forty-second vice president of the United States
- Dennis Rodman, basketball player
- Theodore Roosevelt, twenty-sixth president of the United States

- Elizabeth Taylor, actress
- Martin Van Buren, eighth president of the United States
- Dominique Wilkins, basketball player
- Woodrow Wilson, twenty-eighth president of the United States

The Littlest Gift

There was one surprising advantage to my first asthma attack, but it was entirely due to timing: I was five years old, it was Christmas Eve, and I wanted to see Santa Claus when he came to my house with the presents.

Every previous Christmas Eve, the excitement of the holidays had meant I hadn't a prayer of being able to stay awake and alert enough to see the big jolly man in red. This year, I would have given anything for the relief that sleep would have brought from the exhaustion of not being able to get enough air into my lungs. Still, I held out the faint hope that my wheezing wouldn't be too loud to eclipse the sound of sleigh bells and the hooves of eight reindeer on my roof.

My first asthma attack was precipitated by sitting too close to our church's nativity scene at Christmas Eve mass. To lend a little more authenticity to the scene that year, the church had hauled in bales of real hay and set up some plastic donkeys and horses. My parents thought it would be a harmless treat for me to sit close to the nativity scene so I could see better. I had always loved animals, but I had recently developed quite severe allergies to most of them, including cats and dogs. My parents hadn't counted on the hay itself triggering an allergy—they had logically assumed that if the animals were plastic, I was safe. They were wrong.

Halfway through Christmas Eve dinner, my nose started running, my eyes became red, itchy and watery, and I started coughing. Several hours later, I was in the full-blown horror of an asthma attack, and it was the most frightening thing that had ever happened to me. Every breath was a struggle, and it seemed that the harder I worked to get air in, the harder it became to breathe, and the more tired I became. It was like there was a heavy iron weight on my chest, squeezing all the air out of my lungs and taking away all my strength.

Shortly after midnight on Christmas morning, after a steam bath, hot tea, and allergy medicine had eased my symptoms but failed to cure them, it was clear that neither my mother nor I would be getting any sleep. She decided it was time to go to the hospital. I came out of the bathroom to see her arranging the presents under the tree. The room was dark but comforting, illuminated only by the gentle, cheerful colors of the Christmas tree lights. My eyes moved quickly to the plate of cookies, glass of milk, and carrots for the reindeer. Gone, all of them! I couldn't understand how I'd missed him. I'd been listening so hard. Then, as I watched my mother's quick movements with the logic and clarity of youth that inevitably leads to the first bloom of skepticism, it dawned on me. Maybe Santa Claus hadn't been here at all. I knew he was fast and clever, but how could he have waited until the exact moment when I went to the bathroom to deliver all those presents?

It was time to get this sorted out. "Hey, Mom," I croaked between wheezes, "What are you doing with those presents? Isn't that Santa's job?" I asked accusingly. "Well," she said calmly. "He's so busy that he just needed my help arranging them so they look pretty." I hesitated. This made sense, and she sounded sure of herself. Still, something didn't seem quite right.

"You can pick one present to open now and take with you to the hospital," she said gently but firmly. Still disgruntled at having missed the magical Santa Claus and growing crabbier by the minute, I picked the smallest package from the pile and was surprised when it made a little musical sound. I tore off the wrapping to reveal a miniature keyboard, not much wider or longer than the palm of my hand. I was instantly enchanted, and I did take it to the hospital with me, trying to concentrate on making familiar songs with its lovely delicate tones rather than my wheezing and exhaustion.

The little keyboard has long since lost its sound, but my asthma is much better. To this day, listening to any kind of music calms me in the midst of an attack. And my mother's real gift from that Christmas endures—she still does her best to shield me from disappointments, large and small, which I'm sure will never change.

♥ *Anne Stopper*

What Is Asthma?

Asthma is a disease that affects the airways in and out of the lungs. In a person with asthma, the airways are swollen or inflamed. They are very sensitive, and when you breathe in something irritating, or that you're allergic to, the airways narrow and become more inflamed.

The muscles around the outside of the airways also tighten up, making the airways even smaller. Cells in the airways make more mucus than usual, which also leads to narrower airways. The result of all these changes: less air gets to your lungs, which leads to wheezing, coughing, a feeling of chest tightness, and breathing difficulty. This is called an asthma attack, or episode.

Some asthma attacks are worse than others. In a severe asthma attack, the airways may become so narrow that the body is starved of oxygen, and the result can be deadly.

That is why it's so important to take asthma seriously. If you have asthma, visit your doctor regularly, avoid things that trigger your breathing problems, and take your medicines just the way your doctor tells you to. You'll be able to live life to the fullest and feel your best.

DIAGNOSING ASTHMA

A doctor diagnoses asthma based on a number of things, including your symptoms, family history of asthma and your breathing. As part of the exam, your doctor will use a device called a spirometer to check your airways. The spirometer measures how much air passes through the airways and how fast you can blow air out of your lungs after taking a deep breath. If you have asthma, the results will be lower than normal.

Depending on the results of your physical exam, medical history, and breathing tests, your doctor will figure out how severe your asthma is. The type of asthma you have determines how it should be treated. It's important to remember that a person with any type of asthma—even the mildest form— can still have asthma attacks. The four main categories of asthma are:

- **Mild intermittent (comes and goes)**—Your asthma is not well controlled, you have asthma symptoms twice a week or less and you are bothered by symptoms at night twice a month or less.
- **Mild persistent**—Your asthma is not well controlled and you have asthma symptoms more than twice a week, but no more than once in a single day. You are bothered by symptoms at

night more than twice a month. You may have asthma attacks that affect your activity.

- **Moderate persistent**—Your asthma is not well controlled, you have asthma symptoms every day and you are bothered by nighttime symptoms more than once a week. Asthma attacks may affect your activity.
- **Severe persistent**—Your asthma is not well controlled, you have symptoms throughout the day on most days and you are bothered by nighttime symptoms often. In severe asthma, your physical activity is likely to be limited.

When You First Hear the Word "Asthma"

Hearing from your doctor that you or a family member has asthma may bring on some strong emotions. You may not want to believe it's true. You might be scared, anxious or depressed. Those feelings are all normal.

Once you accept that you or your loved one has asthma, you can start taking steps to control your breathing. Working with your doctor, you will learn how to identify and control asthma triggers and take asthma medicine to prevent asthma attacks. You'll have an asthma action plan to tell you exactly what to do if you feel your breathing start to change.

> The more you learn about your asthma, the more confidence you'll have in your ability to manage any breathing problems that may arise. You'll avoid unnecessary hospital visits, and be able to let go of those feelings of distress.

Allergies and Asthma

While you or your child may have asthma but not allergies, or allergies but not asthma, many people have both conditions together. Eczema (allergic skin inflammation) and hay fever are the two most common allergies that people with asthma have. If you suffer from hay fever and you have asthma, you know only too well the feeling of a runny nose and watery eyes combined with the wheezing and coughing that signal an asthma attack.

Mold, dust mites, animal dander and cockroaches can also cause allergic symptoms in the nose and eyes while causing asthma symptoms in the airways.

Think about . . .
my asthma attitude

These are the things asthma keeps me from doing:

_____

_____

_____

I wish I didn't have asthma because:

_____

_____

_____

If I was never bothered by asthma, I would:

_____

_____

_____

Something I've learned from having asthma is:

_____

_____

_____

The Angry Elephant

An angry elephant is sitting on my chest. When I struggle to breathe, the elephant only presses harder, closing off my airways, making each breath more difficult than the last.

The elephant's name is asthma.

Usually, the elephant leaves me alone. I run around waiting on tables at my restaurant job without getting winded. I play tennis, hike and practice yoga. I laugh and quarrel with my husband and gossip with my girlfriends. Most of the time, I'm just another middle-age woman who worries about money, loves her family, and wonders what it might be like to kiss Brad Pitt.

Without warning, I catch a nasty cold that turns into a stubborn cough followed by a tightness in my chest, and an inability to talk without wheezing. My lungs feel as if they are full of glue.

Removing that elephant off my chest is all that matters. I don't worry about wrinkles or credit card bills or squabbles at my job. Each labored breath is more precious than the last. When my asthma gets out of control, I'm reminded that the nasty elephant is still on my chest. Since I was diagnosed with asthma 20 years ago, I've been hospitalized twice, not counting several emergency room visits and countless sleepless nights gasping for air.

And yet I sometimes still have trouble admitting I have asthma.

Growing up, everyone called me the healthy child, the one who danced through life never out of breath. It was different for my mother and little brother. My mother wore a medical alert bracelet identifying her as an asthma patient. One bee sting could trigger an allergic reaction and an asthma attack. My little brother had to drink syruplike, bitter medicine and sleep in a cloud of vaporized steam to keep his lungs open.

I was the strong, free girl while my mother and brother were imprisoned with sensitive, sick lungs. They had allergies that might trigger asthma while I could rub my face in a cat's fur without my eyes watering. I played all day in a field of flowers and tall grasses without worrying about pollen. Dust only made me sneeze, not wheeze. When I caught a cold, I didn't have to be rushed to the doctor like my brother.

While dealing with their asthma, neither my mother nor my little brother ever complained, or acted sorry for themselves or were afraid it might kill them. They both just accepted that it was part of who they were, like having blue eyes or an outward belly button. I often reflect on my childhood and admire how bravely my mother and brother lived with asthma during a time when there weren't many advanced medications.

I was the one who whined about asthma. Why couldn't we have a cat? Or goose-down pillows? Why did my mother have to spend my seventh birthday party in a hospital bed? Why did we have to cut short our vacation to Canada just because my brother was wheezing?

During my early twenties, I moved away from home and put my family's asthma behind me. I smoked cigarettes, worked in smoky nightclubs, slept on feather pillows in dusty rooms and took my lungs for granted as I always had.

Then, when I was 29, my genetic time clock kicked in. I always was the late bloomer. Part of me was glad I escaped asthma as a child, and the other half of me refused to truly accept the doctor's diagnosis.

I didn't like to tell friends for fear they might view me as "weak." It embarrassed me to use my inhaler in public. I took my doctor's advice and medication haphazardly. I told people I didn't mind if they smoked in my house. I'd wait until that elephant was stomping on me before I'd seek help and then become impatient when the doctor couldn't "fix me" immediately.

I wanted to pretend I was still that little girl with the perfect lungs who only watched other people have asthma. All I could see was what was taken from me and not what was given, the opportunity to take better care of my body.

With age comes many things, but especially the understanding that immortality is reserved for people in white robes with wings. Besides, the mirror won't let me pretend I'm a little girl anymore. Breathing matters more than other people's opinions.

As I inch closer to 50, my angry elephant and I have finally come to an agreement. I take my medications, get plenty of rest, don't smoke, avoid air pollutants and get exercise. I go to the doctor without shame.

Asthma has taught me I must accept my weakness to truly be strong.

♥ *Susanne Brent*

Asthma Triggers

A person with asthma has his or her own set of asthma "triggers." These are things that can set off a reaction in your lungs that can lead to an asthma attack. Triggers can be found indoors or outdoors. Check off the triggers that make your asthma worse:

__ Cold air

__ Tobacco smoke

__ Exercise

__ Wood smoke

__ Perfume

__ Paint

__ Hair spray

__ Other strong odors or fumes

__ Dust mites

__ Pollen

__ Molds

__ Pollution

__ Animal dander (tiny scales or particles that fall off hair, feathers or skin of pets)

__ Common cold, flu or other respiratory diseases

__ Other (fill in here)_____

It's not always easy to figure out what your

triggers are. If you do know what they are, cutting down your exposure to them may help you avoid asthma attacks.

If you don't know your triggers, try picking one or two on the list above and limiting your exposure to them. See if your asthma gets better. This may indicate these are triggers for your asthma.

IN YOUR HOME

Some people with asthma find their symptoms get worse at night. If you're one of these people, try sleeping with air conditioning. Because you keep the windows and doors closed, you're keeping pollen and mold spores outside. Air conditioning also lowers the humidity indoors, which helps control mold and dust mites.

The following are tips for controlling common triggers:

Tobacco smoke. Don't allow smoking in your home. Ask family members and guests to smoke outside. Even better, suggest they quit smoking!

Cockroaches. Small pieces of the insects and their droppings end up in house dust, and from there, into the air you breathe. To get rid of roaches:

- Store food in sealable containers and keep crumbs, dirty dishes and other food cleaned up.
- Fix leaks and wipe up standing water.

- If you choose to use a pesticide, consider baits—they're less likely than sprays or foggers to harm your lungs.

Indoor mold. Bathrooms, kitchens and basements are prime spots for mold when humidity is high.

- Make sure air circulation is good in these areas, and the areas are cleaned often.
- Consider a dehumidifier for the basement—empty the water and clean the container often to prevent mildew.
- Wash foam pillows every week to get rid of mold that may form from perspiration. Dry them thoroughly and change them once a year.
- Check houseplants for mold. You may need to keep plants outdoors.

Strong odors or fumes. Avoid or use very sparingly:

- Perfume
- Room deodorizers
- Talcum powder
- Paint
- Cleaning chemicals

Dust mites. These tiny, microscopic spiders are found in house dust. One pinch of dust may have several thousand mites.

- Put mattresses in dust-proof, allergen-impermeable covers, and tape over the zipper.
- Put pillows in allergen-impermeable covers, and tape over the zipper. Or wash the pillow every week.
- Wash all bedding every week in water that is at least 130° F. Removing the bedspread at night may help.
- Don't sleep or lie down on upholstered furniture.
- Get rid of carpeting in the bedroom.
- Clean up dust as often as you can, using a damp mop or damp cloth. Don't use aerosols or spray cleaners in the bedroom. And don't clean when someone with asthma is in the room.
- To avoid dust on window coverings, use window shades or curtains made of plastic or other washable material for easy cleaning.
- Remove stuffed furniture and stuffed animals (unless the animals can be washed), and anything under the bed.
- Closets are a big source of dust mites. Try putting clothes in a plastic garment bag (not the plastic bag that covers dry cleaning).
- Get a dehumidifier because dust mites like moisture and high humidity.
- Try a vacuum with a high efficiency filter or a central vacuum that blows dust and other allergens outside the home.

Pets and Asthma

It can be devastating to a family to find out that a family member's asthma is triggered by a beloved pet. Dogs and cats can trigger asthma problems, but so can other animals, like birds, guinea pigs or hamsters. Doctors recommend that the pet in question be removed from the home when it triggers asthma, but that's not an easy decision to make. What should you do?

If you do decide to remove the pet, it's important to know that pet allergen remains in house dust and may continue to trigger asthma symptoms even after the pet is gone. Clean the house—especially carpets and upholstered furniture—thoroughly. If you are looking to get a new pet, try tropical fish.

It's also important to explain to children that the pet is being removed for important health reasons. Children in the household who don't have asthma may feel resentful about losing their pet and blame the person with asthma. Explaining that the pet can cause serious breathing problems for a person with asthma may help the child to understand why the family has made this difficult decision.

If you decide to keep the pet, there are measures you can take to help cut down on the amount of allergen that is spread through the house. But no matter what you do, animal allergen will still be in the air and carried on the clothing of people in your home, so you'll still be exposing the person with asthma to allergens.

Ways to cut down on animal allergens in the home include:

- Keeping pets out of the bedroom of the person with asthma and keeping the door closed.
- Keeping pets away from carpets, fabric-covered furniture and stuffed toys.
- Vacuuming carpets, rugs and furniture two or more times every week.

Think about . . .
cutting down on asthma triggers

A big change I can make is to:

_____

_____

_____

An easy change I can make is to:

_____

_____

_____

When I'm cleaning I will:

_____

_____

_____

I'll get rid of:

_____

_____

_____

I'll ask family members to:

_____

_____

_____

The Air Quality Index

Those hazy days of summer can be hard on the lungs of people with asthma. That's because ozone, the primary ingredient of smog air pollution, is very harmful to breathe. Luckily, you can find out at the beginning of each day how bad the air is, and plan accordingly, with the help of a very handy tool—the Air Quality Index, or AQI. This is the system that state and local air pollution control programs use to notify the public about levels of air pollution.

In most cities and suburbs, air pollution levels are measured daily and ranked on a scale of 0 for the cleanest air all the way up to 500 for air pollution levels that pose immediate danger to the public. The AQI further breaks air pollution levels into five categories, each of which has a name, color and advisory statement.

How Do You Find Air Quality Information?

- Air quality forecasts may be included as part of your local weather forecast on TV and radio, or printed in the newspaper. AQI levels are also available online, through local agencies and the U.S. Environmental Protection Agency (EPA) (*www.epa.gov/airnow*).

- State and local air pollution control agencies are responsible for collecting air quality data and reporting the AQI. You can call them for current information if it is not available through the media. A directory of state and local agencies is available from STAPPA/ALAPCO, their national membership association, at *www.cleanairworld.org.*
- The EPA issues year-round AQI forecasts for 46 states plus the District of Columbia. Forecasts include animated pictures of ozone and particle pollution levels superimposed over a map of the United States. The map illustrates how pollution levels change and move throughout the day. It is "real time" information, so you can see current outdoor air quality. The map is available at *www.epa.gov/airnow.*

Breathing to Death

It was stupid. But at the time the whole thing made perfect sense to me. I had convinced myself that I was going to cure myself of asthma.

I used to ask my doctor for a cure. He always laughed at me. I am the kind of person who makes people laugh, so when I asked for a cure, he thought I was joking.

I wasn't joking. When I told the doctor that someday I was going to just throw all the medicine out and let this asthma cure itself, I wasn't joking either. I wanted to get rid of asthma like an old coat. I was tired of sewing on patches. The patches looked ugly and the coat wasn't keeping me warm anymore.

Having had asthma from childhood and having lived through this miracle cure and that miracle cure, I guess I had just overdosed on being a pill-inhaler-steroid-dependent. I was tired of hearing about all the people with "seasonal asthma" who were getting relief from some new pill that was making springtime poetic. I was sick of hearing about people with "exercised-induced asthma" getting relief from some new inhaler used before swimming 900 miles at top speed.

I was having problems sleeping through the night and walking through the supermarket; the new drugs weren't doing a thing for me.

I was living in the nineties. People were jogging to the mall and aerobic kickboxing their way into the twenty-first century. I couldn't get from one end of my house to the other without using an inhaler. And the inhaler didn't always work, so the doctor was pumping me up with prednisone, a drug that was causing me to gain weight. And I was living on the stuff.

Because of my asthma, we moved from New York to Arizona, where, at the time, they said the air was cleaner and drier. In Arizona I might have a better chance at good health. We got off the plane along with a half million other people, and these other people all had cars that helped pollute the desert air and they lived in houses with swimming pools which each added to the overall humidity level. And they told two friends. And so on. And so on. Arizona was not the answer.

I was already in a mild depression from living a life where I had to think about what I could and couldn't do. People with the best intentions were always asking me why I wasn't taking the pill that so-and-so was taking and getting relief from. If so-and-so could win a gold medal in the Olympics, I certainly had no excuses for restricting my activities.

So I threw out my medicine. I threw out the inhalers and the pills. I threw out the breathing machine and the gadget that helped me measure my breathing effectiveness. I threw out the doctor's phone number. I threw it all out.

The fatal error is that I almost killed myself in the process of trying to cure myself. My body shut down totally. I stopped breathing. I was curled up on the floor with my husband screaming into the phone for 911 to send help, with my sons staring down at me, crying, "Don't let Mommy die!"

Then the ambulance came and they got me to the hospital. I was hooked up to machines. The doctors pumped me up with this and that. I don't remember most of it. And three days later in intensive care, my doctor was scratching his head saying, "You were serious?"

The truth was that I was seriously depressed, and no one recognized it.

I'd been putting up that false medicated front for so long that recognizing it might have been impossible. I'd spent a lifetime of sitting away from everyone who was sitting in the grass because the grass made me wheeze. I spent a life of not having friends with pets because I couldn't visit them. I spent a life of avoiding foods and activities and places. We saved for years and went to Hawaii. Everyone went scuba diving. I held the towels. I fretted through two pregnancies of taking life-sustaining medicines in spite of the potential damage to the fetuses. Friends were afraid to take an aspirin for a headache when they were pregnant; I lived on mass quantities of medicines through both pregnancies, worrying constantly of potential side effects the medicines were going to have. Two healthy children later, my asthma kept getting worse.

There was a time when I could predict an attack. Now the attacks were coming without signs. And I was taking a ton of drugs that were helping me mildly, but not enough to allow me a normal existence.

My doctor became wiser after seeing me in intensive care. If he had passed me off to a therapist, I don't think I would have gained control of my asthma and ultimately, regained control of my life. I don't think until this time he quite understood the level of depression that I was suffering because of my asthma. I think I scared him. And more important, I scared myself.

A few weeks after the night in the emergency room, the doctor called me. He told me a new medicine was being released. This time it was my turn to be lucky. It worked.

I'm not a doctor, but I am an expert on my own asthma. And as an expert, it scares me that death can be as simple as a breath away, and it empowers me knowing that I've gained control of my life and my greatest fear.

♥ *Felice Prager*

Take Charge of Your Health Care

While it is up to you to determine the ways to deal with and treat your asthma, having a strong relationship with your doctor will help you make the best choice. Your doctor can help you figure out how to deal with your symptoms and how to work with you to help you breathe easier.

Make a list of your questions before you visit the doctor and feel free to refer to the list during your visit. If your doctor says anything you don't understand, ask to have it repeated. If doctor visits tend to overwhelm you, bring along a friend or relative who can take notes, offer support and help ask questions.

Tell your doctor about:

Any herbs or dietary supplements you're taking. Just because you can buy them without a prescription doesn't mean they're harmless.

Your symptoms. Describe your symptoms: when they started, how they make you feel, what triggers them and what you've done to relieve them.

Your daily habits. Don't be embarrassed—be honest about your diet, physical activity, smoking and alcohol or drug use. Your doctor can't give you the best care if you withhold information.

Ask about:

• **Test results**—how will you find out about

them and how long it will take to get them.

- **Side effects** of any medication you've been prescribed. Are there alternatives? How much will
it cost, how long will it last and will insurance
cover it?

- **How to take the medicine:** what to do if you
miss a dose; if there are any foods, drugs or
activities you should avoid when taking the
medicine; and if there is a generic brand available at a lower price—you can ask your pharmacist these questions, too.

GETTING A SECOND OPINION

There are times when you may not feel comfortable with a particular doctor. Don't dismiss those
feelings. If you don't feel at ease talking with that
person, you may want to consider switching
doctors.

Or you may not agree with your doctor's recommendations. In that case, you should think about
getting a second opinion. Another doctor might have
a different perspective or new options for treatment
and give you new information.

Here are some tips on how to get a second
opinion:

- Ask your doctor to recommend someone
else—either another primary care doctor or a

specialist—for another opinion. Don't worry about hurting your doctor's feelings. If you prefer, you can call a university hospital or medical society in your area for names of doctors.

- Check with your health insurance provider to see if they cover the cost of a second opinion, and make sure the person you're going to is covered under the plan. Find out if you need a referral from your primary care doctor.
- Have your primary care doctor send medical records to the doctor you're seeing for a second opinion so you don't have to repeat any medical tests. Your primary care doctor's office may charge a fee for this service.
- As with your primary care doctor, come prepared to meet the new doctor with a list of questions and concerns.
- Ask this doctor to send a written report to your primary care doctor, and get a copy for your own records.

*"I tell patients, 'If you brought your car
in to the mechanic and you picked it up
and it clunked out of the parking lot,
you'd go back in and demand that it be fixed.
You need to do that with your asthma.'"*

—LeRoy Graham, M.D., pediatric pulmonologist

Beating Asthma

It was my first year at summer camp, and I was
excited and scared, but more important, I was
alone. I had taken a plane to Wisconsin, hundreds
of miles away from my home, to spend three long
weeks away from my parents.

A few days later, I was in love with camp. I
enjoyed all the different activities, from swimming
in the lake to eating with my cabin mates in the big
mess hall.

One day, I was very late to dinner and I was scared
that I would get in trouble with my counselors. I
loved all of them and I desperately wanted to be a
great camper. I dashed out of my cabin, slammed the
screen door and started running across camp. As I
ran I felt my chest start to coil tighter and tighter, but

I was in too much of a hurry to stop and worry about it. As I stopped in front of the mess hall, I noticed there was a squeaky sound coming from my chest and that it was very hard to breathe. As I went into the mess hall and sat down, I just kept trying to ignore it, but my breathing was getting worse.

Finally, I gathered my courage and went up to my youngest counselor, Laura. I sat down on the bench next to her and said, "Laura, I can't breathe." She looked really surprised and I could tell she couldn't quite believe me. She told me to put my head on her lap and concentrate on breathing. But my breathing was getting worse and I was starting to panic.

At last, Laura helped me up and we started walking across camp to the infirmary. As we walked, I vaguely remember Laura talking to me and telling me to keep breathing, but I was so terrified, the walk was a blur. When we got to the infirmary, the doctor put a mask over my face and told me to breathe deeply. Finally I could breathe! When the treatment was over, the doctor sat down next to me and said, "Emily, I think you have asthma, I am going to order you an inhaler and it will be here tomorrow." I was sure he was kidding. Me, have asthma? No way! But he said it was true.

The next day, as I came to realize my fate, I was terrified. Here I was, hundreds of miles from home, and the scariest thing that had ever happened to me was happening without my parents. My counselors tried to be there for me, but I was miserable, and sick too. That summer I spent more time in the infirmary than out.

At last I came home, and my asthma was confirmed through breathing tests. My asthma is now well controlled with the help of steroids, and I have the support I need from my parents and friends. I am so proud of myself, because I know I am beating asthma.

♥ *Emily Bamberger*

Treat Your Asthma

The type of asthma medicines you take depend on how severe your asthma is and other factors. These medicines keep the airways open. Asthma medicines are sold under many brand names and come in many forms, including sprays, pills, powders, liquids and shots. No one drug is best for every kind of asthma or every person. You and your doctor need to work together to find the best medicines and the right amounts for you.

When your asthma is properly treated, it should be controlled, and you should not have asthma symptoms. If you are taking asthma medicine and you still have trouble breathing, don't just assume this is "normal" for you. It's not! Tell your doctor what your symptoms are and when you have them. Then you can work with your doctor to find the right medicine or combination of medicines to keep your asthma under control.

MEDICATIONS

There are two main types of medications for asthma:

Quick relief medicines are taken when your asthma symptoms are getting worse and you may be on your way to having an asthma attack. These medicines start working within minutes to prevent an asthma attack.

You use quick relief medicines only when needed. A common type of quick relief medicine is a **short-acting, inhaled bronchodilator**. Bronchodilators relax tightened muscles around the airways. They help open up airways quickly and make breathing easier. Although these medicines act quickly, they only last for a short time. You should take quick relief medicines when you *first* begin to feel asthma symptoms like coughing, wheezing, chest tightness or shortness of breath. You should always have a quick-relief inhaler in case of an attack. Your doctor may also suggest that you use your quick-relief inhaler before you exercise.

Long-term control medicines are taken every day, usually for a long period of time, to control ongoing symptoms and to prevent asthma attacks. It usually takes a few weeks before you feel the full effects of these medicines. If you have persistent asthma, you'll need long-term control medicines.

• **Inhaled corticosteroids** are the most effective long-term control medications for asthma. This medicine reduces the swelling of airways that makes asthma attacks more likely. Inhaled steroids are recommended for mild, moderate and severe persistent asthma. Your doctor will show you how to correctly use the inhaler. In some cases, steroids are given in tablet or liquid form for a short time to bring asthma under control, or for a longer time to control severe asthma.

- **Long-acting beta-agonists** help control moderate and severe asthma and prevent nighttime symptoms. Long-acting beta-agonists are taken together with inhaled corticosteroids.
- **Leukotriene modifiers** are used either alone to treat mild persistent asthma or together with inhaled corticosteroids to treat moderate persistent asthma or severe persistent asthma.
- **Cromolyn** and **nedocromil** are used to treat mild persistent asthma.
- **Theophylline** is used either alone to treat mild persistent asthma or together with inhaled corticosteroids to treat moderate persistent asthma. People who take theophylline should have their blood levels checked to be sure they are taking a safe dose.

Many people with asthma need both a short-acting bronchodilator to use when their symptoms get worse and long-term, daily asthma control medication to treat the underlying inflammation of the airways that causes asthma.

Think about . . .
my asthma medicines

Here are the asthma medicines I take:

Name	Dose	How often I take it	Why I take it

Side Effects

If you have any of the following side effects, tell your doctor—he or she may change the dose or try a different medicine:

- Sore throat
- Nervousness
- Nausea
- Rapid heartbeat
- Loss of appetite
- Staying awake

Think about . . .
my health checklist

Work with Your Doctor

Go through this checklist before you visit the doctor, and be sure to share your answers with the doctor.

Since my last visit:

My asthma is worse.	___YES	___NO
I've had changes in my home, work or school environment (such as a new pet or someone smoking).	___YES	___NO
At least one time, my symptoms were a lot worse than usual.	___YES	___NO
My asthma has caused me to miss work or school or reduce or change my activities.	___YES	___NO
I've missed any regular doses of my medicines.	___YES	___NO
My medications have caused me problems (shakiness, nervousness, bad taste, sore throat, cough, upset stomach).	___YES	___NO

I've had an emergency room visit
or hospital stay for asthma.   ___YES ___NO

The cost of my asthma treatment
has kept me from getting the
medicine or care I need for my
asthma.   ___YES ___NO

I have increased how often I
take quick-relief asthma
medicine.   ___YES ___NO

I have woken up at night more
often because of my asthma.   ___YES ___NO

Get a Flu Shot

If you have asthma, you should get a flu shot.
The flu, or influenza, can cause an asthma attack
and poses a major health risk to people with
asthma. For some people, a flu-induced asthma
attack is serious enough to require a trip to the
emergency room. A study conducted by the
American Lung Association found the flu shot
will not cause an asthma attack in children and
adults with asthma.

Life Off Stage

The diagnosis was frightening. How could I be so healthy one day and, weeks later, be receiving the news I had asthma? The American Lung Association once said, and to me it is all too true, "If you can't breathe, nothing else matters." I had never felt grateful for my breathing until now.

I wasn't aggressive about seeking medical help. Being a successful, healthy dance studio owner, I believed that I could control most things. I would allow only two or three days away from work, no matter what the illness. I felt irreplaceable. Being dependent, needy and vulnerable for weeks, then months, was a truth I couldn't grasp.

Life now revolved around my nebulizer, a compressor for dispensing inhaled steroids, my many bottles of medicine and wishing life would be as it once was.

Who was I if I couldn't perform my roles as business person, wife, mother, grandmother? What was my purpose? Exhausted continually, I had been forced off the stage of my life.

A trip to a large medical center presented me with my first hope: a doctor who spoke encouraging words about treatments for asthma. She pressed her stethoscope to my chest as I struggled to inhale, lungs burning. The exhale, even without a stethoscope, produced a squeaking, whistling sound, very familiar to me by then. She wrote me prescriptions and we scheduled a follow-up visit.

Time and medication began to restore my breathing and my energy. I still have asthma. But my asthma has made me appreciate more fully life's gifts: I witnessed the birth of my granddaughter on a chilly summer morning in Alaska, I celebrated my birthday with my husband from a hot air balloon, I made sandcastles with my grandchildren, I cheered for my sister as she became a pilot, I loved more deeply than I thought possible.

This life off stage has brought gratitude, an awareness of my blessings and richness far beyond anything material. Today, I live with intention, looking forward, making decisions based on a "no regrets" criteria. I no longer ask myself who I am off stage. The answer clearly lies in who and what I love.

♥ *Vicki Armitage*

Get an Asthma Action Plan!

When you or a family member has asthma, you have a lot to keep track of. That's why every person with asthma needs an asthma action plan. The plan is written by your doctor to help you manage your asthma. It tells you what to do based on changes in your symptoms and your peak flow numbers (see peak flow meter section below).

An asthma action plan is especially important in an emergency. Keep copies of it handy, and make sure it's current. Review it with your doctor at least once a year.

USE A PEAK FLOW METER

To help you measure your lung function, your doctor may give you a handheld device called a peak flow meter to use at home. To use it, you take a deep breath and blow hard into a tube to find out how fast you can blow out. This gives you a peak flow number. You find out your "personal best" by writing down the peak flow number daily for a few weeks until your asthma is under control. The highest number you get during that time is your personal best peak flow. You can compare future peak flow measurements to your personal best peak flow, and that will show if your asthma is under control.

Your doctor will tell you how and when to use

your peak flow meter and how to use your medicine based on the results. The peak flow meter can help warn of a possible asthma attack even before you notice any symptoms. If your peak flow meter shows that your breathing is getting worse, you should follow your action plan.

WHAT'S MY NORMAL PEAK FLOW RATE?

Peak flow rates are usually broken down into three zones: green, yellow and red.

Green Zone:

Eighty to 100 percent of your usual or "normal" peak flow rate means all clear. A reading in this zone means that your asthma is under reasonably good control—just keep following the asthma management program your doctor has recommended.

Yellow Zone:

Fifty to 80 percent of your usual or "normal" peak flow rate means caution. Your airways are narrowing and may require extra treatment. Your symptoms can get better or worse depending on what you do, or how and when you use your prescribed medication. You and your doctor should have a plan for yellow zone readings.

Red Zone:

Less than 50 percent of your usual or "normal" peak flow rate means a medical alert. You may be experiencing severe airway narrowing. Take your rescue medications right away. Contact your doctor now and follow the plan he or she has given you for red zone readings.

We suggest you have a written, easily located asthma action plan in your house. To download the American Lung Association Asthma Action Plan, visit *www.lungusa.org* and type "asthma action plan" in the search box.

ASTHMA ACTION PLAN

Work with your doctor to fill out this information.

General Information:

Name_____

Emergency Contact_____

Phone Numbers _____

Physician/Health Care Provider _____

Phone Numbers _____

Severity of Asthma

__Mild Intermittent

__Mild Persistent

__Moderate Persistent

__Severe Persistent

Triggers

__Colds

__Exercise

__Animals

__Smoke

__Dust

__Food

__Weather

__Air pollution

__Other_____

Exercise

1. Premedication (how much and when)

2. Exercise modifications _____

_____

GREEN ZONE: Doing Well

Peak Flow Meter Personal Best=_____

Symptoms

• Breathing is good

• No cough or wheeze

• Can work and play

• Sleeps all night

Control Medications

Medicine	How Much to Take	When to Take It
_____	_____	_____
_____	_____	_____
_____	_____	_____

Peak Flow Meter

More than 80 percent of personal best or _____

_____

YELLOW ZONE: Getting Worse

Contact physician if using quick relief medicines
more than two times per week.

Symptoms
- Some problems breathing
- Cough, wheeze or chest tight
- Problems working or playing
- Wake at night

Peak Flow Meter

Between 50 to 80 percent of personal best or

_____ to _____

Continue control medications and add:

Medicine	How Much to Take	When to Take It
_____	_____	_____
_____	_____	_____
_____	_____	_____

**IF your symptoms (and peak flow, if used)
return to Green Zone after one hour of the
quick relief treatment, THEN**

__ Take quick-relief medication every four hours
for one to two days

__ Change your long-term control medicines by

_____

__ Contact your physician for follow-up care

**IF your symptoms (and peak flow, if used)
DO NOT return to the GREEN ZONE after
one hour of the quick relief treatment, THEN**
__ Take quick-relief treatment again
__ Change your long-term control medicines by

_____

__ Call your physician/health care provider
  within__hours of modifying your medication
  routine _____

_____

RED ZONE: Medical Alert
Ambulance/Emergency Phone Number:

Symptoms:
• Lots of problems breathing
• Cannot work or play
• Getting worse instead of better
• Medicine is not helping

Peak Flow Meter
Between 0 to 50 percent of personal best or ___

_____ to _____

Continue control medications and add:

Medicine   How Much to Take   When to Take It

_____   _____   _____

_____   _____   _____

_____   _____   _____

Go to the hospital or call for an ambulance if

__ Still in the red zone after fifteen minutes

__ If you have not been able to reach your
    physician/health care provider for help

__ Other _____

Call an ambulance immediately if the following
danger signs are present:

__ Trouble walking/talking due to shortness of
    breath

__ Lips or fingernails are blue

Disney Dreams

I was diagnosed with asthma at a very exciting time in my life. I had just been accepted as a performer at a major theme park in the United States. Now it seemed that my dream was unlikely to come true.

As an athletic college student, my sudden breathing problems came as a big surprise. The road to diagnosis was a bumpy one. At my lowest moment, I could not even walk across my college campus without getting out of breath. I couldn't understand how a seemingly healthy person could develop this kind of chronic disease overnight. How was I ever going to be able to perform in a theme park when I couldn't even walk across campus? It didn't seem possible. I didn't know anybody who had asthma, and I felt very alone. I was referred to a very good physician, who was able to help me start on the path of my new life.

I found out that not only did I have asthma, I also had allergies that triggered my asthma. By getting my allergies under control, I was able to get my asthma under control. I was able to start working out for the first time since I had started school, and it finally seemed like my dream of performing would once again be a reality.

As I geared up for the possibility of being a performer, I engaged in a lot of prayer and soul searching. I worried whether I would be able to handle the physical nature of my new job, especially in light of my new diagnosis. With the help of some good friends at my campus's Catholic Newman Center who supported me during this turbulent time in my life, my family and two very good doctors, my dream is now a reality. I perform in up to three parades a day in the extreme heat, and while having asthma means it is not always easy, it has made my victory that much sweeter.

My new goal for myself is to become more physically active and one day participate in the Danskin Women's Triathlon at Walt Disney World, a feat that seemed impossible even before my diagnosis. When I was first diagnosed with asthma, I would never have dreamed of setting my sights on such a goal. I know now, however, that with a little prayer and determination, I can do anything. Who knows? Perhaps one day I will see you at the finish line.

♥ *Jessica Berger*

When Your Asthma Isn't Under Control

If your asthma doesn't seem to be getting better even though you are taking steps to control it, don't be discouraged. Here are some possibilities to explore with your doctor:

- **Something in my home is triggering my asthma.** Reread the section on asthma triggers in this book, and think about whether any of the common asthma triggers—dust mites, pet dander, cockroaches, mold or tobacco smoke, for example—could be triggering your symptoms.
- **Something in my workplace is triggering my asthma.** Do some of your coworkers also have asthma symptoms at work? Does your breathing improve on weekends or vacations? If so, your doctor can help you figure out what the trigger might be, and if you can avoid it.
- **I'm not taking my medication correctly.** Go over the medication plan that your doctor has given you to make sure you're following it exactly.
- **I'm not using my inhaler the right way.** If you don't use your inhaler correctly, you're probably not getting enough medicine into your lungs. Ask your doctor if you need a spacer, a

device that helps more of the medicine get deeper into your lungs. Your doctor will show you how to use a spacer correctly.

- **I may need to change medicines.** If the medicines you're taking aren't controlling your asthma, you may need to change them. For instance, you may need to take one long-term controller medicine every day to fight inflammation in the lungs, and also take a quick-relief medicine to deal with asthma symptoms.
- **I don't know when my asthma is getting bad.** You may need to use a peak flow meter several times a day to monitor how well your lungs are working. Keeping track of your peak flow can tell you if you may need to take extra medicine or call your doctor. Your doctor will teach you how to use a peak flow meter and how to interpret the results.
- **I may have medical triggers such as GERD (heartburn with reflux) or chronic sinusitis.** Up to 70 percent of people with asthma have GERD compared with 20 percent to 30 percent of the general population. If you have severe, chronic asthma that does not respond well to treatment, you are even more susceptible to GERD. Sinusitis also is common in people with asthma.
- **Maybe I don't really have asthma.** If you've

followed all your doctor's instructions and still are having problems, perhaps you have another illness that acts like asthma. Your doctor may want to do other tests to make sure you really have asthma.

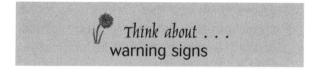

Think about . . .
warning signs

Do you have any of these signs? It might mean your asthma is not under control:

__ My asthma symptoms are occurring more often.

__ My asthma symptoms are worse than they used to be.

__ My asthma symptoms are bothering me a lot at night and making me lose sleep.

__ My asthma is causing me to miss work.

__ My child's asthma is causing him or her to miss school.

__ My peak flow number is low or varies a lot from morning to evening.

__ My asthma medications do not seem to be working very well anymore.

__ I have to use my short-acting, quick relief or rescue inhaler more often. (Using quick relief medicine every day, or using more than one inhaler a month is too much.)

__ I have had to go to the emergency room or doctor's because of an asthma attack.

__ I have ended up in the hospital because of my asthma.

Asthma Can't Smash Olympic Ambitions

I was diagnosed when I was 18, a freshman at UCLA, and we didn't know exactly what was going on. But I was doing a lot of wheezing and had shortness of breath and had been misdiagnosed with bronchitis. Finally, I went to an allergist, and they said I had asthma. And from there, we started working on trying to recognize my triggers, as well as the symptoms.

When I was having the shortness of breath, I thought mainly I was out of shape, and I was afraid UCLA was going to take my scholarship away. And then, once I was diagnosed, I was living in denial. I didn't want to believe that I had asthma, so I wasn't doing the things they were telling me to do to really get my asthma under control.

The key is controlling and managing your asthma, making sure you get your lung function test. It's very important for you to educate yourself on your medication, working with your doctor so you can control your asthma and stop living in denial. After you do that test, go over those results

with your doctor. It could tell you where you are
and then start following a program to start better
controlling your asthma. Because asthma shouldn't
control you. You should be controlling it. And that's
the one thing I had to do, because at one particular
time, asthma was controlling me.

♥ *Jackie Joyner-Kersee*, six-time Olympic medalist,
from National Public Radio interview with Tavis Smiley

Asthma and Exercise

Some people with asthma begin wheezing and breathing harder after they exercise, or after they run up stairs or carry heavy things. This is called exercise-induced asthma.

Unfortunately, many people with exercise-induced asthma simply stop exercising because they want to avoid asthma attacks. But then they become out of shape, and even more likely to have breathing problems when they do anything strenuous.

Don't let asthma stop you from exercising! The benefits of exercise are too great to miss. Exercising reduces your risk of heart disease, helps you lose weight, makes you look and feel great, reduces stress . . . the list goes on and on.

The trick is to choose the kinds of exercise that are least likely to cause breathing problems, and to work with your doctor to see if you need to take medicine before exercising to avoid having an asthma attack.

Signs of exercise-induced asthma include breathing trouble (wheezing, chest tightness, coughing or chest pain) within 5 to 20 minutes after exercise. In some people, asthma symptoms start after they stop exercising. Cold air, air pollution, high pollen counts and colds all can worsen the effects of exercise-induced asthma.

If you think you may have exercise-induced asthma, ask your doctor. He or she can do a breathing test while you exercise to see if you indeed have this problem.

The best activities for people with exercise-induced asthma include

- Swimming
- Walking
- Leisure biking
- Hiking

When exercising outdoors in cold weather, wear a scarf over your mouth and nose so you inhale warm air.

If you enjoy team sports, try those that require short bursts of activity, such as

- Baseball
- Softball
- Volleyball
- Tennis
- Football
- Wrestling
- Short-term track and field events
- Golfing

Treatment

If your doctor determines you have exercise-induced asthma, you may be given inhaled medication to take before exercising. The most common medicine is a short-acting inhaled bronchodilator used fifteen minutes before exercise. If this treatment isn't sufficient, your doctor may consider giving you long-term control medicine to take daily.

🌸 *Think about . . .*
my favorite types of exercise

The type of exercise I enjoy most is_____.

This exercise can bring on
asthma symptoms.   ___YES ___NO

Another type of exercise I can try is_____.

I do a warm-up before
starting to exercise.   ___YES ___NO

I do a cool-down after exercising.___YES ___NO

I've talked to my doctor about
asthma and exercise.   ___YES ___NO

> You should also warm up before
> exercising, and do a cool-down, including
> stretching and jogging, to prevent air in your
> lungs from changing temperature too quickly.
>
> Avoid exercising when you have a cold or other
> respiratory infection, or when it's very cold
> outside. If your asthma is triggered by air
> pollution or pollen, avoid exercising outdoors
> when levels of these irritants are high.

*"He wants to run and jump like any other kid—his
asthma doesn't stop him. He won't quit—he just
gets his inhaler and keeps going."*

—RACHEL G., MOTHER OF AN EIGHT-YEAR-OLD WITH ASTHMA

Camp Catch Your Breath

We arrived at Jackson's Mill, West Virginia, that afternoon not knowing what to expect. We unloaded our suitcases, then my mom went to sign us in at the camp registration table while my grandmother took a reluctant look around.

After we were signed in, we headed into our cabin, picked out beds and made them. "You girls don't have to stay here, you can come home with us right now," my mother said as her eyes welled with tears. "We'll be okay, Mommy," my sister and I replied.

It was our first time at camp. Mandy was nine and I was eight. "Are you sure you'll be okay?" "Yes, Mommy."

So we headed outside. Mom kissed us good-bye and told us she loved us. We started to play with another one of the campers. Mom and Grandma stood by the cabin and watched us play, and the camp director came over and reassured them that we would be all right. So in tears, Mom and Grandma departed.

We were at Camp Catch Your Breath, a little camp held every year at Jackson's Mill for children with asthma. I had enjoyed myself so far, but a little while later I found myself sitting on my bed, a single tear streaming down my face. I missed my mom. But soon enough, I was having a blast with everyone in camp.

By the end of the week, I had had so much fun that I cried because I didn't want to leave. I had also learned so much that week. I found out that my asthma could not limit what I do, that I in fact had the control. I was better able to handle any scary situation with my asthma that arose and all that I owe to the wonderful people who took the time out of their summer to educate children about their asthma.

I returned to camp every year after that. To this day I attend Camp Catch Your Breath, but now as a counselor. Growing up through the program, I felt it was my responsibility to give back to a camp that gave me so much. It's not only something that I love to do, but it's an extremely fulfilling experience to know that you can make a difference in children's lives, by helping them to realize that they are in control of their life and their asthma, and that just because they have asthma doesn't mean that they can't do everything that every other "normal" kid can. They can achieve their dreams.

♥ *Jessica Rogerson*

Asthma in Children

Asthma is the leading chronic illness in children. Fortunately, most children with asthma have mild to moderate problems, and their breathing problems can be controlled with treatment at home. If your child is being kept awake at night, isn't able to participate in their favorite activities like ballet or soccer, or is missing school because of their asthma, then it's not under control—and you need to let your child's doctor know.

In young children, asthma symptoms may be missed. That's because wheezing isn't the only sign of asthma in children. Frequent coughing, inability to keep up with other children during play and unusual irritability also may be signs of asthma.

Children with frequent respiratory infections (such as pneumonia or bronchitis) should be checked by their doctor for asthma. A feeling of tightness in the chest and shortness of breath also can be signs of asthma.

TREATMENT

Your child's doctor will choose medication for your child based on his or her symptoms and test results. Children's asthma medications often are the same as those for adults, but doses are smaller. Children with asthma may need both a quick-relief inhaler if they feel an asthma attack coming on, and daily medication to control their asthma.

Your child's doctor may ask you to help your child use a peak flow meter to help keep their asthma under control. Measuring a child's lung function with a peak flow meter can be very helpful because it may be hard for a child to describe the symptoms.

You will need to take your child to the doctor for regular follow-up visits and make sure that your child uses the medication properly.

Your doctor may recommend a special device to help your child take asthma medication such as a spacer, which makes it easier for a child to use an inhaler, or nebulizer, which delivers medication in a mist that the child inhales. Your doctor will show you and your child how to take the medicine and use any special devices. If you are not completely sure how to use them, ask again!!

Treatment Tips

- If your child uses a bronchodilator inhaler to deal with asthma symptoms, he or she should begin to feel better within five to ten minutes.
- It usually takes one hour for liquid medicines to work. For pills and capsules, the time varies, so check with your doctor or pharmacist.
- Asthma medicines, including corticosteroids, are safe and highly effective if taken in the recommended doses. All medicines can be harmful if they are not taken properly.
- If your child experiences any side effects from asthma medication, call your doctor. If your doctor cannot be reached, reduce the dose by half, or skip the next dose. Do not stop the medicine completely. This may cause the asthma to get worse.
- Asthma medicine taken by mouth should never be taken on an empty stomach. If your child gets nauseous or vomits, try to give the medicine with some milk or food. Be sure to tell your doctor you are doing this because giving the medicine with food or milk can change its effectiveness.
- If the side effects, such as vomiting, do not go away, talk to your doctor about changing the dose or the type of medicine. Vomiting is an urgent danger sign.

- Asthma medicine needs to be adjusted if your child has symptoms (such as wheezing or coughing) with exercise, at rest, at night or early in the morning. Speak to your doctor about changing the dose or type of medicine.
- For "as needed" medicines, give them within five minutes after symptoms begin. It takes less medicine to stop an episode in the early phases of asthma rather than later on.
- If your doctor agrees, give the medicine at the first sign of a cold or influenza even if you don't hear wheezing or coughing. Continue giving medicine until all signs of the cold or influenza are gone.
- Your child's doctor may prescribe medicine to be taken daily to prevent asthma even if your child does not have symptoms. The medicines reduce airway swelling and make it less likely that another episode will occur.

Think about . . .
my child's asthma

I would like help understanding

_____How my child should use the inhaler

_____How my child should use the peak flow
      meter

_____How my child should use the spacer

_____How my child should use the nebulizer

Other questions I have: _____

_____

_____

_____

Think about . . .
my child's asthma symptoms

___ My child coughs, wheezes, has chest tightness or shortness of breath.

___ Colds go right to my child's chest and last much longer than other siblings.

___ My child coughs or wheezes with exercise, play and laughter or during temper tantrums.

___ We have a family history of asthma or allergies.

___ My child misses school because of asthma.

___ Coughing or wheezing keeps me and my child up at night.

My child's asthma triggers are _____

_____

_____

_____

This is how often my child's symptoms happen, and how bad they are:

_____

_____

_____

Take this checklist to your child's next doctor appointment and discuss it with the doctor.

"I want all kids with asthma to know that when
you take care of yourself and your asthma, you can
still run and have fun!"

—SCOTT H., AGE TWELVE

Running on Asthma

Our family doesn't think of asthma as a bad
thing; it's just a fact of life in our house. Both my
sons have asthma; my youngest son, Sydney, has
been a severe asthmatic since he was three months
old. His older brother, Bradley, has asthma, too, but
not as severe. Sure, they'd rather not have it, but
they do. I have always explained to them that having asthma is like having blue or brown eyes; it is
just part of who they are.

I've discussed with both boys that kids can die
from asthma and that is why they have to always
take their medication correctly. They both know the
medications that they have to take and the schedule
for taking them. They also know to pretreat before
playing too hard (sports, tag, running around).

Sydney is the most coordinated, athletic child I
have ever seen. It can be difficult to balance his

athletic gifts with his asthma. He started running before he was nine months old and I was always trying to slow him down for fear of another asthma attack. Sydney would run as fast as he could, stop suddenly and drop to the ground, catch his breath, and then get up and run some more.

One day I was talking with his physician about the balance between running and asthma. He told me that I have to let Sydney be a "normal" child. He has to be able to follow his dreams; we just have to do it with an inhaler in hand. I finally relented and allowed Sydney to join a baseball team when he was four years old. I was so scared, but I just gave him his medication before the start of the game and held his rescue meds in my hand during all the games.

I had never seen my son so happy. He was doing what he loved . . . playing baseball with the other kids on a team. It has been a year since Sydney first played on a baseball team and since then he has taken ice skating lessons, joined a sports club at school, played street hockey with his big brother and cannot wait to join a team again soon.

It is still hard to let him go, but I know that I have to. More important, he feels he can do anything . . . and he can!

♥ *Shari Davis Gonzales*

Coping with Your Child's Asthma

Finding out your child has asthma can produce a range of emotions. You may be relieved to know what's been causing your child distress. Or you might feel overwhelmed thinking that you'll be dealing with a long-term condition, and you wonder how you'll manage if your child has an asthma attack. It's natural to worry, but with time, and experience, you'll feel more confident about dealing with asthma.

Many children handle the news that they have asthma better than their parents do. It's important to keep a positive attitude. Don't let your concern overshadow your child's growing independence. Hovering over children will not help them.

However, there may be times when you have to make decisions that affect their health—such as deciding that your child can't go to a friend's house because their cat can trigger your child's asthma. Simply say no, tell your child why, and don't dwell on it. Getting stuck in guilt won't help your child—or you.

Help children take responsibility for their asthma as they get older. They'll gain pride and self-confidence when they master the day-to-day tasks involved in caring for their asthma. Praise them as they take on more responsibility, and acknowledge that it can be scary for you to let go a little bit. But remember, they will need to learn to care for themselves as they grow.

Preschoolers can:

- Help with peak flow monitoring with close parental supervision.
- Start to find words to describe their symptoms.

School-age children can:

- Perform peak flow monitoring and take medications with supervision.
- Tell parents when they feel an early onset of asthma symptoms.
- Be allowed to play and participate in sports.

Pre-teens can:

- Understand the consequences of failing to manage asthma.
- Have more independence in taking medication, peak flow monitoring and following their asthma action plan.

Some coping tips for parents of children with asthma:

- It's important to remember that with proper medical care, your child with asthma *can* have a normal childhood.

- Realize the impact that your child's asthma is having on his or her siblings. Schedule some one-on-one time with your nonasthmatic children. Plan a special activity, or cook their favorite meal once in awhile—it's a way of showing them that they're special too.
- Don't downplay the stress that dealing with your child's asthma causes. You're coping with fears of your child's illness, visiting the doctor and managing your child's medication regimen. You need to get enough sleep and eat nutritiously. Otherwise, you won't have enough energy for yourself or your family.
- Get sources of support—friends, family and local support groups for parents of children with asthma. Contact local groups such as the American Lung Association, Allergy and Asthma Network/Mothers of Asthmatics and the Allergy and Asthma Foundation of America to find out what information and help they can offer you.
- Read as much as you can about asthma—the more you know, the easier it will be for you to deal with your child's health in a confident and calm manner.

READER/CUSTOMER CARE SURVEY

CEAG

We care about your opinions! Please take a moment to fill out our online Reader Survey at **http://survey.hcibooks.com**. As a **"THANK YOU"** you will receive a **VALUABLE INSTANT COUPON** towards future book purchases as well as a **SPECIAL GIFT** available only online! Or, you may mail this card back to us and we will send you a copy of our exciting catalog with your valuable coupon inside.

First Name | MI. | Last Name

Address | City

State | Zip | Email

1. Gender	4. Annual Household Income	6. Marital Status	Comments
☐ Female ☐ Male	☐ under $25,000	☐ Single	
2. Age	☐ $25,000 - $34,999	☐ Married	
☐ 8 or younger	☐ $35,000 - $49,999	☐ Divorced	
☐ 9-12 ☐ 13-16	☐ $50,000 - $74,999	☐ Widowed	
☐ 17-20 ☐ 21-30	☐ over $75,000		
☐ 31+			

3. Did you receive this book as a gift?
☐ Yes ☐ No

5. What are the ages of the children living in your house?
☐ 0 - 14 ☐ 15+

Do you have your own Chicken Soup story that you would like to send us?
Please submit at: **www.chickensoup.com**

🌼 Think about . . .
how I feel about my child's asthma

My concerns about my child's asthma are

_____

_____

_____

A time when I wasn't sure what to do about my
child's asthma was _____

_____

_____

_____

I'd like to improve the way I handle my child's
asthma by _____

_____

_____

*"I can see his symptoms before
he can even feel them."*

—Barbara Beroff, mother of a ten-year-old son with asthma

Like Mother, Like Son

I left the pediatrician's office with an infant carrier in one hand and a brand new nebulizer in the other. I had presented a brave face in the doctor's office, but tears welled up as I walked to my car. My beautiful, angelic baby boy was what I had prayed he wouldn't be—a wheezer. I secured the baby in the car and sat in the driver's seat and cried. Like me, my baby was destined for a life of "can'ts"—can't spend the night with a friend with a pet, can't run barefoot through a grassy field, can't leave home without an inhaler.

My son's medication regimen was new to me. As we began his treatment plan, which included a daily maintenance drug, I learned more about new medications and how far science has come to control asthma symptoms. Control asthma? I thought you just rolled with the punches—or rather the coughs and wheezes. I was using a store-bought inhaler and used it when I needed it, which was a lot more than the directions on the package recommended.

A few months later, two back-to-back asthma attacks sent me to the emergency room, sweating and in danger. The physician treated me and said, "It would be really senseless for you to die of an asthma attack. Asthma is so treatable. But left untreated, there is no resuscitating the overworked lungs." I thought of my husband and baby waiting for me at home. *Okay, Lord, I understand now. I have to plan to be around for a long time, to see my children grow up and have children of their own. I have to lead by example for my son about how to live with asthma. It is up to me.*

I went home and called a specialist. After meeting with him, all my excuses fell away. New mom, too tired, too busy—I had no good excuse for not taking charge of my health.

Today, my son and I each take a daily maintenance drug. I have done my best to avoid our "triggers" and am prepared to treat symptoms quickly. My son is young enough that I pray that he will outgrow his asthma. But if he doesn't, that's okay. We can live, and live well, with asthma.

♥ *Shawn Scott McSwain*

How to Head Off
a Child's Asthma Attack

Every child with asthma has a built-in early warning system that signals when an asthma attack is impending. Even if your child is not old enough to tell you how they feel, you can learn to look for the signs before the symptoms get bad.

WARNING SIGNS

- Cough
- Unusual paleness or sweating
- Anxious or scared look
- Flared nostrils when the child tries to get some air
- Pursed lips breathing
- Fast breathing
- Vomiting
- Hunched-over body posture; the child can't stand or sit straight and can't relax
- Restlessness during sleep
- Fatigue that isn't related to working or playing hard
- The notch just above the child's Adam's apple sinks in as they breathe in
- Spaces between the ribs sink in when the child breathes in

WHAT TO LISTEN FOR

- Coughing when the child has no cold
- Clearing of the throat a lot
- Irregular breathing
- Wheezing, however light
- Noisy, difficult breathing

HOW TO LISTEN

Put your ear to the child's back and your hand on his or her chest. You'll feel the chest go up as the child inhales, drawing in air, and you'll feel the chest go down as the child exhales, releasing air.

- Listen for squeaking or any unusual noises. They may mean asthma, bronchitis or a chest infection. Only a doctor can tell for sure, so regard any noisy breathing as a signal that help may be necessary.
- If the child is having symptoms and there are no chest sounds, call your doctor immediately.

WHAT TO DO IMMEDIATELY

Reassure the child by your tone of voice, your attitude of being able to manage, your confidence. All those qualities are catching. Your child will take cues from you and relax.

- If the doctor has recommended a medicine when signals appear, use it. (Don't give the child a special dose unless the doctor said to).

- Encourage normal fluid intake. Drinking too much may actually hurt, not help.

EMERGENCY SIGNS

Call your doctor or get emergency medical care if your child exhibits any of these signs.

- Wheeze, cough or shortness of breath gets worse, even after the medicine has been given time to work. Most inhaled bronchodilator medications produce an effect within five to ten minutes. Discuss the time your medicines take to work with your child's doctor.
- Child has a hard time breathing. Signs of this are:
  — Chest and neck are pulled or sucked in with each breath.
  — Struggling to breathe.
  — Child has trouble walking or talking, stops playing and cannot start again.
  — Peak flow rate gets lower or does not improve after treatment with bronchodilators or drops to 50 percent or less of your child's personal best.
  — Lips or fingernails are gray or blue. If this happens, GO TO THE DOCTOR OR EMERGENCY ROOM RIGHT AWAY!

Think about . . .
my child's asthma action checklist

__ I know the signs of a possible asthma attack in my child.

__ I know what peak flow readings signal a possible attack.

__ I know what medications to use if my child shows signs of breathing trouble.

__ I know how to use the medications.

__ I know where the medications are kept.

__ I know where my child's asthma action plan is.

__ I have the phone number of my child's doctor posted where it is easily seen.

__ I know the name and location of the nearest hospital.

God Knew What I Could Handle

My son Kevin was born premature 12 years ago. I had him when I was 30 weeks into my pregnancy. We had many obstacles to overcome. I never imagined that asthma would be my biggest one.

Kevin was diagnosed with asthma nine years ago. I had no idea that asthma would have such an impact on our lives. I am a divorced mother of three. My other children are 20 and 14. Asthma has affected all of our lives tremendously.

Asthma requires many sacrifices. Each day I pack medicines and a nebulizer machine to go to school with Kevin. When we want to go for an outing, I have to be totally aware of weather and environmental surroundings. When I visit other people, I have to make sure that they don't have pets and no one in the home smokes. Vacations require a lot of preparation. I have to make sure that I inform the doctor. I always have to know where the closest hospital is.

I used to feel that I was being punished because

of the endless nights that I spend awake, the hours that I have to worry about him during the day and the amount of days that I have to miss from my job. And I can't give my other two children the same amount of attention that they deserve.

Then I realized I wasn't being punished.

I feel special because I was chosen to have a child with asthma. It takes a special parent to handle all the obstacles that come along with asthma. I now feel privileged, because God knew what I could handle. When I see Kevin smile or he hugs me I know that I was chosen.

Kevin still misses about 25 days a year from school because of asthma (less than half the number of days he used to miss) and has remained on the honor roll for the last seven years. When he was nine, Kevin was able to play in the snow for the first time in his life. Even more exciting was the news we just received that Kevin is now well enough to join the basketball team. He has achieved his lifelong dream.

♥ *Renee Hall-Freeman*

Asthma at School

The best way for you to be sure that your child's asthma will be well controlled during school is to communicate with your child's teacher, school nurse and physical education teacher. Here's what you'll need to do:

- **Write down your child's asthma and allergy triggers** (such as exercise, pet dander or specific foods). Give the list to teachers, coaches, nurses and other grownups who will be in charge of your child during the school day.
- **Give the school staff a written list of your child's medications.** Include dosages and instructions about when the medications should be taken.
- **Give the nurse emergency medications** along with written instructions for how to respond to an asthma attack or allergic reaction.
- **Provide a list of emergency phone numbers** including your child's doctor.
- **Talk to the school staff about your child's asthma warning signs.**

HOW ASTHMA-FRIENDLY IS YOUR SCHOOL? A CHECKLIST

Children with asthma need proper support at school to keep their asthma under control and be fully active. Use the questions below to find out how well your child's school helps children with asthma.

	YES	NO

1. Is your school free of tobacco smoke at all times, including during school-sponsored events? ___   ___

2. Does the school maintain good indoor air quality? Does it reduce or eliminate allergens and irritants that can make asthma worse? Check if any of the following are present: ___   ___
   ___Cockroaches
   ___Dust mites (commonly found in humid climates in pillows, carpets, upholstery and stuffed toys)
   ___Mold
   ___Pets with fur or feathers
   ___Strong odors or fumes from art and craft supplies, pesticides, paint, perfumes, air fresheners and cleaning chemicals

3. Is there a school nurse in your school all day, every day? If not,   ___   ___
   is a nurse regularly available to help the school write plans and

YES   NO

give the school guidance on
medicines, physical education,
and field trips for students
with asthma?   ___   ___

4. Can children take medicines at
school as recommended by their
doctor and parents? May children ___   ___
carry their own asthma medicines? ___   ___

5. Does your school have a written,
individualized emergency plan for
each child in case of a severe
asthma episode (attack)? Does the ___   ___
plan make clear what action to
take? Whom to call? When to call? ___   ___

6. Does someone teach school staff
about asthma, asthma management
plans and asthma medicines?   ___   ___
Does someone teach all students
about asthma and how to help a
classmate who has it?   ___   ___

7. Do students have good options
for fully and safely participating
in physical education class and
recess? (For example, do students ___   ___
have access to their medicine
before exercise? Can they choose ___   ___
modified or alternative activities
when medically necessary?)   ___   ___

If the answer to any question is "no," your child may face obstacles to good asthma control at school. Talk to the principal and school nurse about making your child's school more asthma-friendly. If you need help, contact one of the organizations listed in the Resources section of this book.

"Anyone with asthma knows the fear of not being
able to breathe—it's the rest of the world that
needs to understand."

—DEBRA W., MOTHER OF TEEN WITH ASTHMA

Asthma at Sixteen

My name is Jessica and I was diagnosed with asthma at the age of six. Here I am now at the ripe age of 16, 10 years later looking back at the ups and downs I've been through growing up with asthma.

Now to someone who doesn't have asthma nor has any knowledge of the disease, this probably would seem like some exaggeration and that asthma is just a ploy for attention or as a gym teacher once put it, "just an excuse," but asthma is a problem that affects millions of children every day.

Today, people are more understanding now that asthma is, in fact, seen as a serious issue, and that it does make seemingly simple activities difficult for a child, such as a game of tag with friends or going out in winter to build a snowman.

I've realized as I've gotten older that it's become

sort of a joke with my friends. They sort of kid about it or call me "wheezer" every once in a while. But when it comes down to it, any time I get out of breath or begin to have a problem with my asthma around my friends, they are always the first to notice and offer help: "Are you all right? Do you have your inhaler with you?"

With all the knowledge I have gained, I am in better control of my asthma, but sometimes it gets the best of me and I panic. But I am lucky to be surrounded by such caring and understanding individuals.

Whenever I feel like my asthma is winning, I just remind myself that I am in control of my asthma and that I can achieve anything I set my mind to. My asthma can't stop me from achieving my dreams.

♥ *Jessica Lynn Blazier*

Asthma Throughout Your Life

There are certain times in a person's life that asthma presents special challenges: the teen years, during pregnancy, and later in life.

TEENS AND ASTHMA

The teenage years can be the worst time to feel different. And that's just how asthma can make teens feel. They may feel uncomfortable having to take medicine or using an inhaler or peak flow meter in front of friends.

Teens with asthma may encounter tough situations—deciding whether to decline an invitation to the house of a friend who has pets that can trigger an asthma attack, or having to sit out a team practice on a day when asthma symptoms are flaring up.

Some teens with asthma may end up avoiding physical activity altogether for fear of having an attack in front of others. Others may use asthma as an excuse to get out of gym class or other activities they don't want to do. What's especially dangerous is when teens forget—or refuse—to take their asthma medicine to prevent or control breathing problems. That can lead to a trip to the hospital if a teen's asthma gets out of control.

The goals for teens with asthma are to

- Understand their disease
- Have a simple asthma action plan
- Feel in control of their lives
- Realize that asthma doesn't define who they are or limit them

If you're a parent of a teen with asthma, it's important to realize that asthma may affect your child's self-esteem. You need to be aware of the possibility that your teen is minimizing asthma symptoms or avoiding taking asthma medication in order to appear just like his or her friends.

Being a parent is never easy, but parenting a teen with asthma has its own special challenges—trying to make sure teens are following their asthma action plan, while giving them the independence to make decisions about their own health.

Some parents of teens with asthma may find it's useful to make a contract with their teens that outlines an asthma management plan and offers rewards and consequences.

You are more likely to avoid confrontations about your teen's asthma if you talk with your teen about what he or she can do to take control of their breathing. Think about what you've been saying—have you been heavy on restrictions and limits, emphasizing what your teen can't do because of asthma?

Instead, accentuate the positive—talk about what your teen can do. Give as much responsibility as you think your teen can handle. Emphasize that now that your teen is older and more independent, it's time to be more responsible for his or her own health. Talk to teens about what can happen if their asthma isn't managed properly and remind them that controlling their asthma will allow them to do the activities they enjoy. Then trust your teen to take medicine at the right time, in the right way. He or she is sure to appreciate your confidence in his or her ability to manage his or her own health.

Offer support and encouragement by

- Allowing your teen to meet with the doctor alone. This will encourage your teen to become more involved in his or her own asthma care.
- Encouraging your teen to meet other teens with asthma so they can offer one another support.

Think about . . .
your teen's asthma

My teenager's feelings about asthma are _____

_____

_____

_____

Problems I've encountered in trying to help my
teen manage asthma are _____

_____

_____

_____

Something that's worked in helping my teen deal
with asthma is _____

_____

_____

_____

I wish my teenager with asthma would_____

_____

_____

_____

Asthma and Pregnancy

If you're pregnant and have asthma, it's especially important for you to stick to your asthma action plan—for the sake of your health as well as your baby's.

It's understandable that a woman with asthma may wonder whether it's okay to take medicine. Studies have shown that most inhaled asthma medications are safe for pregnant women. If you take asthma pills, talk to your doctor about whether you can switch to another medication during your pregnancy.

The good news is that women whose asthma is well controlled during pregnancy have a very good chance of having a normal pregnancy and a healthy baby. Uncontrolled asthma, on the other hand, can lead to a decrease in the amount of oxygen in the mother's blood, which means a decrease in oxygen for the fetus. This can affect fetal growth, because the fetus needs a constant supply of oxygen for normal growth. Uncontrolled asthma can lead to premature birth and a baby with low birth weight.

As soon as you find out you're pregnant, talk with your doctor about your asthma medications and whether they are appropriate and safe to use during pregnancy.

Important facts about asthma and pregnancy include:

- Some women find their asthma gets better during pregnancy, some find it gets worse and others find it stays the same. If your asthma changes, your doctor will adjust your medicine as needed.
- Asthma tends to get worse in the late second and early third trimester of pregnancy. If your asthma is well controlled during pregnancy, you are very unlikely to have asthma troubles during labor and delivery.
- Most women with asthma can perform Lamaze breathing techniques without any trouble.
- Talk to your doctor about getting a flu shot. Influenza is especially dangerous for people with asthma.
- If you smoke, now's the time to quit! Smoking may make your asthma worse, and it directly affects the health of your growing baby. Also avoid being around other people's smoke— secondhand smoke can trigger your asthma and affect your baby, too.

OLDER ADULTS AND ASTHMA

Developing asthma in adulthood can be a big surprise. Some adults who develop asthma remember having had breathing problems as children, which went away, but came back later in life. Others develop asthma for the first time when they are older.

Sometimes an older person can have asthmalike symptoms such as wheezing that actually are the signs of another lung disease. Other lung diseases that cause similar problems are bronchitis and emphysema, especially in people who smoke. Heart disease can also cause breathing problems.

DRUG INTERACTIONS

If you're an older adult with asthma, there's a good chance you're taking medication for other health conditions as well. Some drugs may cause problems for people with asthma. Tell your doctor what medicines you are taking for other health problems. Don't forget to include alternative medicines and vitamin supplements. And remind your doctor about your asthma every time you get a new prescription. Keep an up-to-date list of all the medicines you take. Carry the list with you.

Drugs that may affect asthma include

- **Blood pressure and heart drugs.** Some people with asthma find that their asthma gets worse when they take certain blood pressure drugs such as beta-adrenergic blockers (such as propranolol, nadolol and timolol), or ACE inhibitors.

- **Pain relievers.** Some people with asthma may have breathing problems if they take aspirin, acetaminophen, ibuprofen or naproxen. Such drugs include many drugstore cold remedies and pain remedies.

TREATMENT TIPS

- If you're taking medications for several different conditions, work with your doctor to simplify your medication program as much as possible. Perhaps you can combine medications or use alternate ones that will have the same desired effect.
- Be sure your asthma action plan is written down, and give a copy to someone else—a family member, friend or neighbor.
- If you're having trouble using an inhaler because of arthritis, tell your doctor. If you don't use the inhaler correctly, you're not getting the correct dose. Ask your doctor whether you can use a breath-controlled inhaler, or a special device for inhalers for people with arthritis.
- Some asthma medications increase heart rate. If you feel an increased heart rate, be sure to tell your doctor.
- If you're taking oral steroids, you'll need regular checkups so your doctor can monitor you

for any signs of diabetes, hypertension, glau-
coma, cataracts and osteoporosis.

• Ask your doctor about getting an annual flu
shot and a pneumonia shot (which may be
given every five years to adults 65 and older).

Think about . . .
my doctor's visit checklist

__ Tell my doctor if I've had any change in asthma symptoms since my last visit.

__ Get written instructions on all my asthma medicines—how often to take and what dose.

__ Get written instructions on what to do when my asthma symptoms get worse.

__ Ask the doctor to show me how to properly use my inhaler and/or spacer device.

__ Ask for a peak flow meter and instructions on how to use it to monitor my lung function.

__ Bring medications and peak flow records with me to each visit.

__ Tell my doctor if I've gotten any new prescriptions from any of my other doctors since my last visit.

__ Tell my doctor if I've had to go to the emergency room since my last visit.

My Asthma Friend

I was just over 40 when I was first told that the breathlessness I had been experiencing was asthma. At first, it didn't really strike me as anything too serious. I would take my two different inhalers and I would be fine.

The trouble started when my doctor arranged for me to attend his asthma clinic at our local county hospital. As I walked into the waiting area, there didn't seem to be anyone there under 70 years of age.

I sat there looking around me, thinking everyone looked old and ill. There was frequent coughing, wheezing and I suddenly saw my future before me and was horrified. I began to realize that asthma was something to be taken seriously.

Following that visit, I read up on the different kinds of asthma and the treatments. I found out that, fortunately, my asthma was not too serious and mainly it was a question of getting it under control with the correct medication.

I went to two more of the clinics and hated each

one. At the second one, one of the older gentlemen introduced himself as Ben and tried to make conversation with me. He seemed to have trouble breathing and it was difficult to follow what he was saying. I had little to say to poor Ben; all I wanted was not to end up like him. I was still the youngest person there and after my third visit, I told my doctor I was not going to any further sessions.

For a few months, I had my medication adjusted here and there and was getting on fine. Then, I got a terrible head cold; it lasted for two weeks and went from my head into my chest. I developed a bad wheezy cough that I had never really had before and my asthma was awful. I had to inhale four or five times to get any kind of relief.

I stayed out of work, but one day my husband was working out of town and, feeling a little better, I went into town for some shopping. I was coming out of a shop when I started to cough. I couldn't stop and my wheezing got so bad that I remember collapsing on to the sidewalk gasping for breath, my inhaler useless in my hand. I heard people say, "Call an ambulance, she is choking. . . ."

That was when a calm voice said, "No, an ambulance will take too long, she's having an asthma attack. Help her over to my car, I'll drive her to a doctor." Someone argued and the man said, "I am an asthmatic, she needs to get to a nebulizer as soon as possible. The doctor's office is not far away."

I remember getting into the car, still trying to breathe and in a state of panic. He told me, "Calm down, breathe slowly, let your inhaler do the work."

I did as he said and he drove me the five minutes to the doctor's office. As soon as we got there, he rushed in and people came out to help me. I was soon attached to the nebulizer, the mask over my face and starting to breathe again. The doctor explained that my asthma was pretty well controlled but that getting a really bad chest cold may always be more of a problem, and might require additional medication.

"You were lucky your friend was there and had the sense to bring you straight in to the nebulizer. Waiting for an ambulance would not have been a good idea," he said. "He said you panicked a little. The reason for going to the asthma clinic was to help you cope with that kind of situation."

I nodded. "I'm sorry, I just felt uncomfortable at the clinic. You said my friend—I was so distressed, I don't really know who the gentleman was."

"His name is Ben Patterson. You probably met him at the asthma clinic. He is a wonderful old gentleman. He has bad asthma but never lets it get in his way, still takes long walks, goes off abroad on vacation. He is so eager to help people who are first diagnosed and may think that their world has come to an end. Wasn't he at the clinic when you were there?" he asked me. "Yes, I think he was," I said, not willing to admit I had brushed aside the help of this man who had probably saved my life.

I cried when I told my husband about it later and said, "I must find out where he lives and go and thank him," I said. "Why don't you thank him by going along to the next clinic and listening to what he has to say?" Eric suggested.

I did exactly that. I apologized for how I had responded the first time and thanked him for saving my life. Ben and I became firm friends; he had traveled all over the world and had endless tales to tell of his adventures. He was one of the most interesting people I had ever met and he gave me so much good advice about my asthma. "Accept that you have it, get it under control and get on with your life. If you have to make adjustments around it, then do so, but don't let it have the upper hand in what you can and cannot do, you decide!"

When Ben passed away, some years ago now, there were so many people like me at his funeral. I had met most of them through Ben, and Eric laughingly refers to them as "Your asthma friends." We still talk about Ben and try to pass on to others what this lovely man taught us.

♥ *Joyce Stark*

Traveling with Asthma

People with asthma and their families love vacation time just as much as anybody else. But having asthma means needing some extra preparation before going on a trip.

Here are some tips for having a vacation where you can breathe easy:

MEDICATIONS

- Bring your asthma action plan with you!
- Bring a list of medications that includes the prescription refill number, the name and phone number of the doctor who prescribed it, and the dosage (all this information should be on the medicine's original label).
- Pack not only the amount of medicine you think you'll need, but also a backup quantity just in case you end up staying longer or need extra for any reason. Pack your medication in your carry-on luggage just in case your checked luggage gets lost.
- If you have an emergency epinephrine injection kit for allergic reactions, bring it with you.

EQUIPMENT

- Bring your peak flow meter along with the chart to record results.

- If you use a nebulizer, bring it along. Portable nebulizers are available that can be plugged into the cigarette lighter in a car.
- If you are traveling abroad, make sure you have an electrical current converter for the nebulizer.
- If your asthma is triggered by dust mites, you may want to bring your own allergy-proof pillow or mattress cover.
- If you'll be by yourself in unfamiliar surroundings, consider wearing a medical alert-type necklace or bracelet.

HEALTH INSURANCE

- Ask your doctor for recommendations for an asthma specialist at your destination, or contact the local state medical society at your vacation spot for recommendations.
- Call your health insurance company to find out what they will cover in another state or country, and whether your plan will cover doctor and hospital visits where you are going.

OTHER TRAVEL TIPS

- Ask for a smoke-free hotel room.
- If you're traveling by car, run the air conditioner or heater, with the windows open, for at least ten minutes to reduce mold and dust mites in the car.

If your asthma is affected by pollen or pollution, travel with the car windows closed and the air conditioner on.

While all airplanes within the United States are smoke-free, that's not true for international travel. Ask for a smoke-free flight, or if that's not available, ask for a seat that's as far away as possible from the smoking section.

If you'll be staying with friends or family, explain your or your child's asthma triggers. It may not be a good idea to stay with a family with pets, or with a smoker unless that person agrees to smoke outside during your stay.

If you're camping, be aware that cold air and wood fires may trigger asthma.

Think about . . .
planning my trip

For my next trip I'd love to travel to _____

_____

_____

_____

I'll need to find out these things about potential
asthma triggers at my destination: _____

_____

_____

_____

Potential problems that might arise from traveling to this place are _____

_____

_____

_____

Possible solutions are_____

_____

_____

_____

*"With changes in my medication and
asthma management, I've been able to
train to run a marathon."*

—CHRIS T., SCHOOL NURSE

I'm Breathing!

Breathing—how often I took it for granted when
I was young. Sure, I had frequent colds and
wheezing breaths, but I never knew that I had
asthma. At the age of 44, I had my first life-threatening asthma attack. I resisted being put on prednisone, because I didn't want to gain weight. I just
would not believe that I could die. I was revived on
the floor of my physician's office with four alarmed
doctors hovering over me. It took four shots of
prednisone to save my life and three weeks of high
doses of oral prednisone. I don't know which was
worse, almost dying or the lingering weeks of
recovery.

In the last 15 years, I have discovered just how
precious I am, especially to my family. I have been
blessed with the devotion of my daughters, as they
keep their vigilant watch over me when I am desperately ill. They have shared their thoughts and

dreams with me and have made me laugh and cry.

My asthma has given me something else very precious. It has given me time. Time—the one rare ingredient that the rest of the world can't seem to find. If only there were more hours to the day, days to the week, weeks to the year, then there would be enough time. The more hurried the world becomes, the less time it can capture. I am blessed. I have plenty of time. I can walk slowly on the good days, and I can see more of what I missed when I didn't take the time. I can write the things that are nearest and dearest to my heart.

The most remarkable gift I have received, however, is an inner peace. I no longer rush through the good things in life. I seize the opportunity to watch the blazing sunset from beginning to end. I meet the rosy dawn in the mountains where I live, with a song in my heart as the sun chases away the ribbons of the night. I am thankful for every breath, knowing that my Creator holds each one in His hand. I see the love in my husband's eyes when he looks at me, knowing within those dark green depths that he has never looked upon anyone so lovely.

There are new treatments for asthma, and I am on an aggressive regimen. In 1994, my pulmonologist promised me that within 10 years there would be new drugs approved that would be nothing short of miraculous. I didn't believe her, yet it has become a reality for me. My serious asthma attacks are now fewer and farther apart. Thankfully, they are shorter and less life-threatening. I make certain to keep up with the latest treatments, and I keep a good working relationship with my doctor, based on mutual respect and trust.

At 59, I am in charge of my asthma, instead of my asthma being in charge of me. Asthma has given me many things. It has given me strength and determination, so that I will never let it conquer my spirit. I am thankful for each new day. I have faith. I have hope. I have love. I am precious. Life is beautiful, because I'm breathing!

♥ *Jaye Lewis*

Breathing Easier

By following all the steps outlined in this book and working closely with your doctor, you should be well on your way to breathing easier. You know your asthma, or your child's asthma, is under control if you can say

__I don't cough.

__I don't have shortness of breath or rapid breathing, wheezing or chest tightness.

__I don't wake up at night because of asthma symptoms.

__I can engage in normal activities including play, sports and exercise.

__My child isn't absent from school or activities because of asthma.

__I'm not missing any time from work because of asthma.

__I haven't had any asthma episodes lately that require a visit to the doctor or emergency room.

__My lung function is normal or near normal.

__I only need my reliever medication less than twice a week.

One thing I've always wanted to do but never have because of asthma is _____

_____

Now that you have a plan to keep your asthma under control, there's no excuse. Now you have it in writing, it's up to you to make it happen. Enjoy!

Resources

Allergy and Asthma Network—Mothers of Asthmatics, Inc.
2751 Prosperity Avenue, Suite 150, Fairfax, VA 22031 (1-800-878-4403; 703-385-4403, Fax: 703-573-7794) Newsletter: The MA Report *http://www.aanma.org/*

American Academy of Allergy, Asthma & Immunology
611 East Wells St., Milwaukee, WI 53202 (1-800-822-2762; 414-272-6071) *http://www.aaaai.org/*

American College of Allergy, Asthma and Immunology.
85 W. Algonquin Rd., Suite 550, Arlington Heights, IL 60005 (847-427-1200) *http://www.acaai.org/*

American Lung Association
For your local chapter or a respiratory therapist: 1-800-LUNG-USA. National Headquarters: 61 Broadway, 6th floor, New York, NY 10006 (212-315-8700) *http://www.lungusa.org/*

Asthma and Allergy Foundation of America
1233 20th St. NW, Ste. 402, Washington, DC 20036 (1-800-7ASTHMA; 202-466-7643, Fax: 202-466-8940) Newsletter: *The Asthma and Allergy Advance http://www.aafa.org/*

Centers for Disease Control and Prevention
To learn more about asthma, visit *www.cdc.gov/asthma.*

Environmental Protection Agency (EPA)
To learn more about controlling indoor asthma triggers, visit *www.epa.gov/asthma*. Call the EPA's Indoor Air Quality Information Line at 1-800-438-4318 to order free materials about indoor asthma triggers. To learn more about the Air Quality Index (AQI), visit *www.epa.gov/airnow.*

National Heart, Lung, and Blood Institute Information Center, National Institutes of Health
PO Box 30105, Bethesda, MD 20824-0105 (301-592-8573) *http://www.nhlbi.nih.gov/*

National Jewish Medical and Research Center
1400 Jackson St., Denver, CO 80206 (303-388-4461) *www.NationalJewish.org/*

Lung Line. 1-800-222-LUNG.
Talk to a nurse and request printed information be sent to you. Library Information Pathfinder on the Web and in the Library; a multilevel approach to information access from the Gerald Tucker Memorial Medical Library.

Supporting Organization

✝ AMERICAN LUNG ASSOCIATION.

The American Lung Association is the oldest voluntary health organization in the United States, with a national office and constituent associations around the country. It works to prevent lung disease and promote lung health. Lung diseases and breathing problems are the primary causes of infant deaths in the United States today, and asthma is the leading serious chronic childhood illness. Smoking remains the nation's number one preventable cause of death. Lung disease death rates continue to increase while other major causes of death have declined.

The American Lung Association has long funded research to discover the causes and seek improved treatments for those suffering with lung disease. They are the foremost defender of the Clean Air Act and laws that protect citizens from secondhand smoke. The Lung Association teaches children the dangers of tobacco use and helps teenage and adult smokers overcome tobacco addiction. They help children and adults living with lung disease to improve their quality of life. With the generous support of the American public, the American Lung Association is *"Improving life, one breath at a time."*

For more information about the American Lung Association or to support the work they do, call 1-800-LUNG-USA, or visit the Web site at *http://www.lungusa.org.*

Who Is Jack Canfield, Cocreator of
Chicken Soup for the Soul?

Jack Canfield is one of America's leading experts in the development of human potential and personal effectiveness. He is both a dynamic, entertaining speaker and a highly sought-after trainer. Jack has a wonderful ability to inform and inspire audiences toward increased levels of self-esteem and peak performance. He has coauthored numerous books, including *Dare to Win, The Aladdin Factor, 100 Ways to Build Self-Concept in the Classroom, Heart at Work* and *The Power of Focus.* His latest book is *The Success Principles.*

www.jackcanfield.com

Who Is Mark Victor Hansen, Cocreator of
Chicken Soup for the Soul?

In the area of human potential, no one is more respected than **Mark Victor Hansen**. For more than 30 years, Mark has focused solely on helping people from all walks of life reshape their personal vision of what's possible. His powerful messages of possibility, opportunity and action have created powerful change in thousands of organizations and millions of individuals nationwide. He is a prolific writer of bestselling books such as *The One Minute Millionaire, The Power of Focus, The Aladdin Factor,*and *Dare to Win.*

www.markvictorhansen.com

Who Is Norman H. Edelman, M.D.?

Norman H. Edelman, M.D., is vice president for Health Sciences and professor of medicine at SUNY Stony Brook University. He is also the chief medical officer for the American Lung Association.

Dr. Edelman is a member of the Association of Physicians, American Society for Clinical Investigation, American Federation for Clinical Research and the American Thoracic Society. In January of 1990, he was appointed to membership to the National Commission on Sleep Disorders Research. He is a fellow of the American College of Physicians and the American College of Chest Physicians.

A former member of the Editorial Boards for the Journal of Applied Physiology and the American Review of Respiratory Diseases, Dr. Edelman has published extensively in the field of pulmonary diseases and control of breathing. In 1990, he was named recipient of a MERIT award for the National Institutes of Health, National Heart, Lung and Blood Institute. He is the author of the *American Lung Association's Family Guide to Asthma and Allergies.*

A graduate of Brooklyn College, Dr. Edelman received his M.D. degree from New York University.

Dr. Edelman has appeared on a number of national news programs, including *Good Morning America, CBS Evening News, Dateline NBC* and *MSNBC.* He has been interviewed by several major newspapers and wire services, including *USA Today, Washington Post, Los Angeles Times, Reuters* and the *Associated Press.*

Who Is Celia Slom Vimont (writer)?

Celia Slom Vimont is a health and medical writer. A graduate of the Columbia School of Journalism, she has written for magazines, newspapers and wire services for both consumers and physicians. The former Director of Editorial Services for the American Lung Association, Celia served as in-house editor for books on asthma and smoking cessation for the association and continues to write about a variety of lung health issues. She is the writer of two previous books in the *Chicken Soup Healthy Living* series, *Weight Loss* and *Menopause*. Celia lives in New York City with her husband and son.

More Chicken Soup

Many of the stories in this book were submitted by readers just like you. If you would like more information on submitting a story, visit our Web site at *www.chickensoup.com.* If you do not have Web access, we can also be reached at:

Chicken Soup for the Soul®
PO Box 30880, Santa Barbara, CA 93130
Fax: 805-563-2945

Contributors

Vicki Armitage is the owner of Vicki's Dance Studios in central Louisiana and has been a guest on the Oprah Winfrey Show. Much change and time away from her roles have provided insight for her life's second journey and the memoir she will someday write. *vckilyn@aol.com*, 3215 Parkway Drive, Alexandria, LA 71301.

Emily Bamberger is 15 years old and lives with her mom, dad, her little sister, Elissa, and dog, Bindi, in Kansas City. Emily has had asthma for three years. She developed it at summer camp.

Jessica Berger is a college student from Missouri currently studying psychology. A published poet, featured in the 2005 edition of *Who's Who in Poetry*, this is Jessica's first short story to be published. Jessica's plans include authoring fiction and nonfiction.

Susanne Brent was born in Chicago and earned a journalism degree from Metro State College in Denver. Susanne now lives in Phoenix, Arizona, with her husband, Ed, and her sweet, old dog, Buddy. Recent publishing credits include nonfiction in *Cup of Comfort for Christmas* and *A Matter of Choice: 25 People Who Transformed Their Lives.*

Shari Davis Gonzales is the mother of two beautiful boys: Bradley, age nine, and Sydney, age five. She and her husband, Mike, have been married for 16 years and live in sunny Redington Beach, Florida. Shari has been an active volunteer with the American Lung Association for five years.

Renee Hall-Freeman is a choir director and public speaker. She resides in Columbus, Ohio, with her husband William and sons, Charles and Kevin, and daughter Kenee. Reneé can be contacted at *hallfreeman@aol.com.*

Jaye Lewis is an award-winning writer who believes that where there is breath there is hope. A severe asthmatic, Jaye looks for reasons to rejoice in the most difficult of circumstances. You can read more of Jaye's inspirational stories on her Web site at *www.entertainingangels.org.* E-mail Jaye at *jayelewis@comcast.net.*

Shawn Scott McSwain is a working mom who lives with her husband, Tom, and son, Jack, in Raleigh, North Carolina.

Felice Prager is a freelance writer from Scottsdale, Arizona, with credits in local, national and international publications. In addition to writing, she also works with adults and children with moderate to severe learning disabilities as a multisensory educational therapist.

Jessica Rogerson is 16 years old and lives in West Virginia with her mother, father, sister, two dogs and two cats. Jessica enjoys reading, listenning to music, playing piano, writing and drawing. She also enjoys being in 4-H. She plans to one day be a member of the FBI.

Joyce Stark lives in North East Scotland and works for the Community Mental Health. Her hobby is writing about people around her and those she meets on her travels in the United States. She has completed a series to introduce very young children to a second language and is currently working on a travel journal of her trips to "Small Town/Big City America." E-mail her at: *joric.stark@virgin.net.*

Anne Stopper is a freelance journalist and former Fulbright scholar to Ireland who lives and works between the United States and Ireland. Her articles have been published in newspapers from Washington, D.C., to northeastern Pennsylvania. She has also worked in broadcasting for National Public Radio's flagship news program *Morning Edition.*

Permissions

Also Available

Chicken Soup African American Soul
Chicken Soup Body and Soul
Chicken Soup Bride's Soul
Chicken Soup Caregiver's Soul
Chicken Soup Cat and Dog Lover's Soul
Chicken Soup Christian Family Soul
Chicken Soup Christian Soul
Chicken Soup College Soul
Chicken Soup Country Soul
Chicken Soup Couple's Soul
Chicken Soup Expectant Mother's Soul
Chicken Soup Father's Soul
Chicken Soup Fisherman's Soul
Chicken Soup Girlfriend's Soul
Chicken Soup Golden Soul
Chicken Soup Golfer's Soul, Vol. I, II
Chicken Soup Horse Lover's Soul
Chicken Soup Inspire a Woman's Soul
Chicken Soup Kid's Soul
Chicken Soup Mother's Soul, Vol. I, II
Chicken Soup Nature Lover's Soul
Chicken Soup Parent's Soul
Chicken Soup Pet Lover's Soul
Chicken Soup Preteen Soul, Vol. I, II
Chicken Soup Single's Soul
Chicken Soup Soul, Vol. I-VI
Chicken Soup at Work
Chicken Soup Sports Fan's Soul
Chicken Soup Teenage Soul, Vol. I-IV
Chicken Soup Woman's Soul, Vol. I, II

Available wherever books are sold • For a complete listing or to order direct:
Telephone (800) 441-5569 • Online www.hcibooks.com
Prices do not include shipping and handling. Your response code is CCS.

Your Case is Hopeless

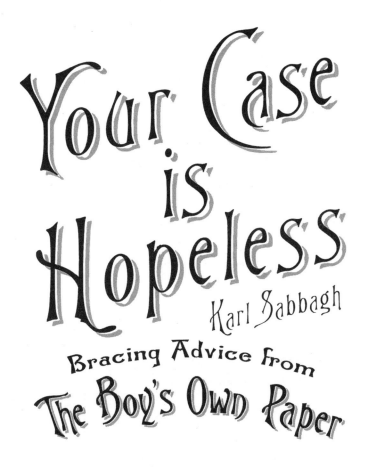

Your Case is Hopeless

Karl Sabbagh

Bracing Advice from The Boy's Own Paper

JOHN MURRAY

First published in Great Britain in 2007 by John Murray (Publishers)
An Hachette Livre UK company

1

Editorial material © Karl Sabbagh 2007

The right of Karl Sabbagh to be identified as the Author of the Work
has been asserted by him in accordance with the Copyright, Designs and
Patents Act 1988.

A CIP catalogue record for this title is available from the British Library

ISBN 978-0-7195-2472-1

Typeset in Walbaum Book Regular

Printed and bound by Clays Ltd, St Ives plc

John Murray policy is to use papers that are natural, renewable and recyclable
products and made from wood grown in sustainable forests. The logging and
manufacturing processes are expected to conform to the environmental
regulations of the country of origin.

John Murray (Publishers)
338 Euston Road
London NW1 3BH

www.johnmurray.co.uk

CONTENTS

Author's Note

One unfamiliar feature about the *Answers to Correspondents* in the BOY'S OWN PAPER is the fact that the original queries are not given, only the answers. Usually, however, it is possible to infer what the questions were about from the answers, though I have included one section in the book where I cannot easily make such inferences but where the answers on their own are thought-provoking.

Usually, answers were preceded by the names or pseudonyms of the writers. I have generally omitted these names, unless they were necessary to understand the answers.

Most of the answers were related to specific topics of interest to boys and I have collected them together as the basis for the chapters of this book. But some answers, usually the longer ones, provide general information that is either surprising, interesting or mysterious. I have organised these answers as 'Miscellanies', which separate the more topic-oriented chapters.

All the answers are quoted verbatim, apart from six words I have inserted into one of the 'Miscellanies' for sentimental reasons. Sometimes, in the accompanying text, I name 'the Editor' as the author of the answers even though it is clear that several different B.O.P. writers helped with the task of answering the deluge of letters that arrived each week.

The valiant work of transcribing and organising more than 1,200 answers into a database to allow for selection and arrangement was carried out by my daughter, Bella Sabbagh, to whom I am very grateful.

Chapter 1

=X=

'BEWARE POOR IMITATIONS'

The birth of the B.O.P.

No one would have predicted the success of the Boy's Own Paper, a publication for boys first published by the Religious Tract Society in 1879 as an antidote to the evil influence of so-called 'Penny Dreadfuls'. These periodicals and cheap books printed bloodthirsty tales of robbers, cannibals and demon barbers, and were very popular with the boys of England at the time, as they had been for the previous forty years.

In its early issues, the Editor of the Boy's Own Paper made clear where he thought the new magazine stood in the market-place:

> We certainly aim to keep the Boy's Own Paper far ahead, in point of real merit, of any of its competitors, though we fear that all boys have not gumption enough to appreciate the vast difference between journals merely filled with improbable stories written to order by people who have never seen, and know little or nothing about, what they profess to describe, and a paper like our own, in which both writers and artists occupy the highest place in public estimation, and are recognised authorities on the subjects which they respectively treat.

(The Boy's Own Paper was never modest about its own fine qualities.)

When the idea of a new paper for boys was first raised, any idea of trying to find out what boys wanted – such a modern approach – was entirely absent. The Religious Tract Society had been in existence for eighty years and its General Committee included a Bishop, a Doctor of Divinity, four clergymen and eight 'Gentlemen'. In 1878 they discussed the idea of 'providing healthy boy literature to counteract the vastly increasing circulation of illustrated and other papers and tales of a bad tendency'.

But what sort of stories can counteract thrilling and lurid tales like *Sweeney Todd, Highwayman Bob* or *The Skeleton Bride* and still be appealing to boys? As it turned out, there didn't seem to be a problem. A story called *Nearly Eaten,* by James Cox, R.N. about a professor on the island of Haiti who was pursued by a horde of voodoo-worshipping cannibals, was a follow-up to a previous story by the same author, called *Nearly Garotted.* And both of these were published in the new BOY'S OWN PAPER.

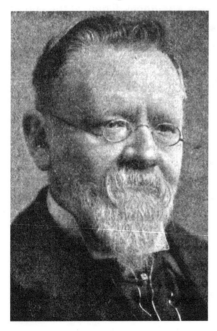

The robust tone of the magazine's stories and articles was set by a man called George Andrew Hutchison, who was appointed to edit it, although because he was rather young, a stripling of thirty-seven with a hint of the working class in his background, he was only called sub-editor, working to an older and more experienced man. But he was editor in all but name, and we can get an idea of the approach he decided to adopt from a remark he made to one of the Secretaries of the Society, that the new magazine would only be a success if it 'appealed to boys and not to their grandmothers'.

Having been appointed, Hutchison was to face endless battles with the Committee, because of his reluctance to include excessive moralising and the Committee's suspicion of writing – particularly fiction – that was designed to appeal to boys' appetites.

The project that the Religious Tract Society approved was more than just a weekly magazine. From the beginning, the BOY'S OWN PAPER was what we would today call a 'brand'. The weekly issues were reissued monthly, as four or five bound together, with an orange cover and several pages of advertisements. Often, the monthly part contained a glossy plate, sometimes in colour and sometimes folding out to reveal Uniforms of the British Army, Flags of All Nations or British Sea Anemones. Then, at the end of the year, all fifty-two issues were bound together and sold as the *Boy's Own Annual*, with two additional special numbers that had appeared during the year, a Summer Number and a Christmas Number. As the fiction serials became so popular, they were then republished by the R.T.S. as B.O.P. books

The success of the magazine, which was clear from the first few weeks, was partly due to Hutchison's eye for quality, which was shown in the people he selected to write. Like some good editors, he 'couldn't write for toffee', as he said himself, but he certainly knew how to spot and improve good writing by others. The very first item in issue No. 1 was by Talbot Baines Reed, a twenty-seven-year-old whose story, *My First Football Match*, set in the fictional public school of Parkhurst, was so well-written and realistic that the B.O.P. regularly received requests from captains of sport at real public schools challenging Parkhurst at football or rowing. Reed had not even been at a public school himself, but that didn't stop him continuing to write thrilling school serials in the BOY'S OWN PAPER, such as *Fifth Form at St Dominic's* and *Adventures of a Three-Guinea Watch*, which were eventually published as extremely successful books. (All of these were produced while he was simultaneously working on a magnum opus called *History of the Old English Letter Foundries, with Notes Bibliographical and Historical on the Rise and Progress of English Typography.*)

A later editor has described the typical BOY'S OWN PAPER hero as 'a boy with strength of character, able to stand up well to risks and temptations, strong and courageous in his actions, a Christian in his daily life, considerate towards friends and fellows, courteous to girls and elders – but neither smug nor pious'.

The first issue also began the serialisation of *From Powder Monkey to Admiral, or The Stirring Days of the British Navy,* and a rather less obviously stirring tale called *Jack and John, Their Friends and Their Fortunes*. Not only did this lack the temperature-raising title, but it was also by a *woman*, Mrs Eiloart. During its early years, the B.O.P. showed the typical Victorian attitude to girls and women that had been taken in by most boys and men with their mother's milk, if that isn't a contradiction.

The masthead on the front cover of the first issue of the BOY'S OWN PAPER showed the words of the title surrounded by symbols of boyhood, such as pets, sports gear and a stamp album.

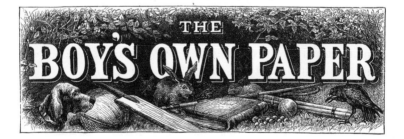

It was designed by Edward Whymper, the conqueror of the Matterhorn, who had lost four members of his expedition on the descent. There was a generally macho feel to all the editorial team, who often had military or naval ranks or let drop hints of sporting prowess. (Even the B.O.P.'s draughts correspondent had a rank – Captain Crawley, 'author of *Manly Games for Boys*, etc, etc', – and a later volume had an article on 'Mr. Arthur Feather, Ventriloquist to the British Army'.) Another contribution in the first issue was by Captain Matthew Webb, first man to swim the English Channel, whose adventurous spirit was to get him drowned four years later while attempting to swim across the rapids at the foot of Niagara Falls for a prize of £12,000, about £2,000,000 in today's money. Webb's first-person account was typical of the non-fiction coverage in the magazine. Another personal story in an early issue was *Adventure with Grizzlies*, by 'the late J.K. Lord, F.Z.S' – how had he become late, I wonder?

In addition to the fiction and the first-person encounters, the B.O.P. included many articles on sports, including archery, athletics, fishing and cycling, as well as the highly popular football and cricket, with contributions from W.G. Grace, who was related by marriage to one of the B.O.P. staff. One of the articles in the first volume was called – rather strangely to modern eyes – *About Football and Other Balls*.

Hobbies were another strong point. Unlike the 'Penny Dreadfuls' which concentrated on fiction, the B.O.P. presented boys with a wide range of pursuits to keep their idle hands from doing the Devil's work. (Although when those hands succumbed, many of them then held a pen to write to the B.O.P. to ask for guidance – see Chapter 3.) Some of the hobbies and pastimes would have required a small engineering workshop to achieve, and even *The Telephone and How to Make It,* in an early issue, called for skills and materials which would stretch many a boy at the time and made demands which would certainly be beyond the 'poorest boys' the magazine sometimes claimed to appeal to.

Then, making up the rest of the magazine, there were regular articles on pets and nature study, as well as competitions and jokes, and the occasional homily about Christian behaviour, such as *A Trick and Its Result:*

> A Lad, for a trick, pointed with his finger to the wrong road when a man asked him which way the doctor went. As a result, the man missed the doctor and his little boy died, because the doctor came too late to take a fish-bone from his throat. At the funeral, the minister said that 'the boy was killed by a lie, which another boy told with his finger.' Probably the lad did not know the mischief he had wrought. Of course he never meant to kill the boy when he pointed the wrong way. He only wanted to have a little fun, but it was fun that cost somebody a great deal. We ought never to trifle with the truth.

Each number was sixteen pages long. The print was very small, and I calculate there were about 24,000 words a week to be commissioned and edited, along with the various illustrations and diagrams that went with the text. Arthur Haydon, the editor after Hutchison – who retired at seventy – remembers being astonished at the system that had been set up to deal with the mass of material required. He found that all B.O.P. copy was kept in tea-chests, with one for each week of the year and other chests for the monthly issues, the Summer and Christmas Special and the Annual volume. These chests were hauled round the office on trolleys to whoever was dealing with a particular issue. Haydon noticed that the chests were all marked B.O.P., not particularly surprising until he discovered that the initials were left over from the tea-chests' former function and stood for Broken Orange Pekoe. (It may be this that triggered a B.O.P. riddle about tea-chests, featuring the Latin phrase *Tu doces*, which means 'Thou teachest'.)

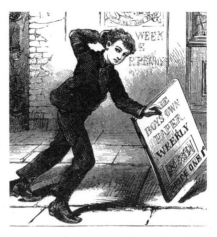

There was a true story told by a later editor that because Hutchison himself was not a particularly pugnacious person, he was unwilling to confront the regular stream of visitors to the B.O.P. offices who wanted to complain, sometimes forcibly, about the rejection of their contributions. So when such callers turned up and asked for the editor, one of the packers from the shipping department, a massive man and a boxer in his spare time, known as the 'Fighting Editor', was summoned and turned up breathing heavily, which was usually enough to settle the matter.

Five years after the B.O.P. began publication, the R.T.S Committee was still concerned that the magazine wasn't evangelical enough, but Hutchison was determined that that way boredom lay. The Committee passed a critical resolution in April 1884 that was read out to Hutchison. Part of it said:

> The proportion of fiction is on the whole excessive, leaving insufficient space for other articles, such as travels and adventure in real life, papers in history, and in the biography of the wise and the good, which would be useful in forming character, as well as affording pleasant reading. Especially the Committee feel that that it is due to the character of the Society and to the best interests of their youthful readers to give more prominence to Christian truth and influence ...

There is no record of Hutchison's response to this, other than the fact that the magazine showed no discernible change in policy and the circulation continued to soar, until it was estimated in the late 1880s to be selling over half a million copies a week, with a readership, therefore, of at least a million.

Of course, the stories and articles in the early numbers of the BOY'S OWN PAPER are period pieces now, even though some of the best fiction writing, by writers like Jules Verne, is sometimes read in book form today. But one regular feature of the magazine, which emerged without fanfare on page 160 of the first volume, was headed simply *Correspondence*, and over the first twenty years of its publication it provided a panorama of all the things that puzzled boys, and sometimes girls, about life in the late Victorian world.

In the first issue of the B.O.P., readers were invited to write in with queries on any topic: 'Our best endeavours will be given to reply to correspondents, who are requested to write as briefly and legibly as possible, and to put no questions requiring private answers.'

Because, as the Editor never tired of pointing out, the magazine went to press six weeks before it appeared on the bookstalls, there was no evidence of any response to this invitation for about three months. Then, in the twelfth issue, the very first answer was given, to 'H.E. Jack and others', who bought the magazines every week but were worried about missing out on coloured plates that were issued only with the monthly edition.

> We have carefully considered your difficulty, and have thus arranged for it. At the end of the year, all the coloured plates, frontispieces, etc., now published only with the monthly parts, will be issued in a sixpenny packet. Buyers of the weekly

numbers will thus find themselves at no disadvantage in regard to binding their papers in volumes.

Now, if the rest of the correspondence was of a similarly banal nature, there would be slim pickings for today's reader among the ten thousand or so letters published in the first decade of the paper's life, but in fact embedded in those pages is a wide-ranging social portrait of late Victorian boyhood, in which answers about hobbies, pets, nature study, careers and even the queries about the magazine itself, gave

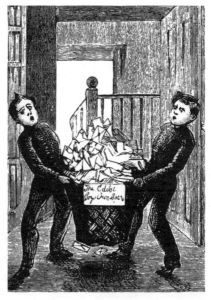

clues to the wider social issues that faced Victorian society.

Already, three months after starting publication, the B.O.P. was feeling the pressure that comes with success. In a reply to several correspondents, the Editor wrote:

> We cannot possibly undertake to reply privately through the post, willing though we might be to oblige by doing so; and even the sending of a stamp or stamped envelope will not constitute an obligation. Will our readers kindly try always to bear in mind that what may be quite practicable in dealing with hundreds, or even thousands, must be something vastly different when it is a question of a quarter of a million; and the number of our readers, all of whom have of course an equal claim on us, can hardly be far short of that now.

The rest of this book gives just a small sample of the thousands of answers to correspondents that were published in the first dozen years or so of the B.O.P.'s existence. Early on, the Editor was compelled to warn the boys that only a few of the thousands who wrote each month would get an answer:

We have again to remind our readers that the letters received are overwhelming in number, and only those the answers to which would convey information useful to the boy public can receive attention. Also that no answer can appear in print in less than six weeks. It is for ailing animals we feel most. Advising for these is in most cases practically useless, as they must be dead or well long ere that time expires. Taking our general run of correspondents, we might class them as follows – (1) the sensible lad who really is in some quandary, and sees no way out of it except appealing to his friend the Editor. (2) The boy who writes when his pet is sick. The obviously best plan for him is to consult, where possible, a local vet. (3) The boy who asks questions that have been answered over and over again, as food for thrushes, rabbits, or mice. Let him read back, or consult our DOINGS. (4) The boy who encloses a stamp, and asks for a reply by post. It cannot be done. Lastly – (5) The boy who writes for writing sake. Now, we do not complain even of these, only they must not expect us to fill up valuable space in replying to them here.

– oOo –

READER, CONSTANT READER, SUBSCRIBER, WELL-WISHER, ETC. – Your inquiries are doubtless all received, but you are so numerous as to be practically anonymous. How many times are we to tell you that such signatures are chosen by the score, and that we never take any notice of the letters so signed? Most of your questions you can answer for yourselves, and many of them would almost seem to be put with an intention of poking fun. Use your initials; put anything you please, as terrible and inappropriate as you like, and we will answer you – but forty 'Constant Readers' in a day! How *can* we assist you? Speaking generally, we do not think much of your handwriting. We know of no cure for freckles or red faces, and when you are introduced to a young lady, 'How do you do?' is as nice an opening to conversation as 'Good morning?' We have heard of a young man who, having been duly introduced, didn't speak a word for nearly ten minutes, when he suddenly blurted out, 'Do you like mashed turnips?' We should hardly advise you to emulate *that*!

– o O o –

E. E. DARIENT – wonders why he has written many times and has not got an answer to his question, 'What subjects should I study to know as much as I should know?' You may rest assured, DARIENT, that you ought to know a great deal more than you ever will know, and that not a subject exists on which you will ever know enough.

– o O o –

We have often said that it is impossible for us to reply to questions through the post. In the untidy scrawl we have received from you we find no less than sixteen ques-tions, which would take something like six weeks to answer fully.

– o O o –

When we have time, we will. We just counted the batch which contained your letter, and there were three hundred and forty-nine separate epistles!

– o O o –

We regret extremely that you have never asked us any questions that have been worth answering, and cordially congratulate you on hav-ing discovered the fact for yourself. And now suppose you try again?

– o O o –

We have no space here for answers to so many and such lengthened inquiries. It is well, as a general rule, to show your acuteness, but it does not always do to cross-examine an editor – through these columns.

– o O o –

AN OLD SUBSCRIBER – What an idea you must have of the corre-spondence of a paper like this, to suppose that we have kept your little bits of paper among our archives! Look at page 48 and endeavour to realise the fact that

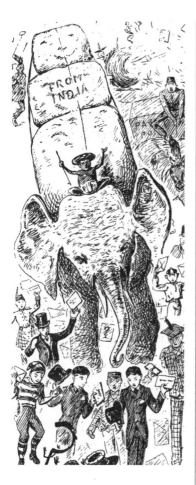

your letter, when it was opened, got mixed with those in the bundles on the elephant's back!

– oOo –

G. E. ABBOT – There, we have put your name in full as you desire. Looks pretty in print, doesn't it?

– oOo –

As 'a constant reader from the commencement' you must have seen that what you ask for has already been done to an extent unattempted by any other periodical, and you can refer to your back numbers for the information. Like a good many other constant readers, your queries betray your inconstancy!

– oOo –

RABBITS. THE BATH. KNOCK-KNEES. INCREASING THE HEIGHT, &c. – Kindly read back. If we kept on answering these queries every week, we should have not tales nor illustrations either.

– oOo –

If a correspondent asks for the nearest Marine Office, or any other office, and does not give his address, his letter is not answered. Your present letter has no address; probably your former letter was on the same plan? Perhaps you will send a third, and explain how we are to tell you the nearest place to nowhere!

– oOo –

Address the Secretary, Science and Art Department, South Kensington, W. It would be as well for you to improve your spelling. 'Dear Idiotor' is not a pleasing commencement.

– o O o –

A READER FROM THE FIRST (and a very careful reader he must be, to judge from his letter): 'Dear Editer. Would you please tell me how many hairs there are on an ordinary cats back as I perticularly want to know. Please whats the best sot of book to read because I want to be an auctioner were can I get it, and how much would it be please?' Now, boys, here is a chance for you! You might as well take the query off our hands, and send us in the 'lot' to be knocked down by the auctioneer! Going! Going!

– o O o –

A READER FROM THE FIRST – An inquiry on your behalf has brought on us quite an avalanche of information as to cats, blacks, and backs, and black cats' backs, most of it singularly novel, and just a little ironical. H. J. W., for instance, says: 'Get the square root of the number of hairs on the cat's

tail, and divide it by the number of the cat's teeth. Subtract from this the circumference of the feline animal multiplied by the square of its cubical content in inches,' and, then perhaps you will quickest arrive at the desired result by following the unfeelingly rude advice of SOBRAON, 'extract the root of your eye-tooth, use it as a multiplier, and immediately hold your jaw.'

– o O o –

For the hundredth time we tell you and other boys – and please to imagine us talking through a speaking-trumpet – that we go to press six weeks before date of issue, and that therefore answers can hardly be expected before the seventh week. What good, then, can accrue from asking advice about a dying dog or canary, or the weather next Sunday, or anything else that needs immediate reply?

– o O o –

We are unable to reply in next issue, as in the first place next issue went to press more than a month ago, and in the second, we really cannot make out what you mean. Perhaps our readers may help us. 'In your next issue give me what information you can upon Mamuls, where they are found at present time, and I want to know whether they were called wholly Elephants, or have they wings on.'

– oOo –

We have also received letters from ATF., 'MATCHBOX' (no); P.T. (any schoolbook will tell you); H.M. (the sentiment is better than the poetry); G. (a matter of taste); REX (the best remedy for biting the nails is to leave off doing it ...); B. (Buckfastleigh); S.U.G.H., AGAMEMNON, ROGER, A.M. and very many others. Your requests shall be borne in mind. More than this we cannot promise.

– oOo –

Your card was addressed simply 'Editor of BOY'S OWN PAPER'; it came to hand all right, but should you write again it would be better for the convenience of the postal authorities, if you cannot find room for the name of the street, to at least put 'London' in the address. Even 'England' would give the postmaster some inkling of the intended destination of your letter.

– oOo –

We really cannot undertake to name and price coins. Why do you not take the trouble to read what is put on every letter-box? *You must not send coins through the post unless you register them.* We have had to pay eightpence on each of your letters.

– oOo –

Please address your letter in the usual way next time – at least, you might put the stamp in front. Your style may be curious and amusing, but it gives a good deal of trouble to sorters and postmen. We give the inscription on your envelope as an example to other correspondents of how not to do it: 'Paid behind. Dear Postman, – If this should cross your path kindly take it to that much worried official called the editor of a paper known to the world as the BOY'S OWN PAPER, who hath his abode at 7 x 8 Row Paternoster backwards. By one who has said this will go to the blindman's office, a would-if-he-could-be comedian. Tootongsombla.'

– oOo –

We have no space here to give you advice about boxing, but we should very much like you to send the twopence we had to pay owing to your having boxed your letter without stamping it. The quickness of the hand doubtless deceived the eye.

– oOo –

J. EWART LITTLE – The most useful thing for an apprentice in a mercantile office is an elementary knowledge of our postal regulations. For instance, if you put a used half-penny stamp on a letter, and fancy that you will not be found out, you are mistaken, and the friend you have favoured with your correspondence will have to pay twopence for your little dodge – which we had to do, O Little!

– oOo –

CONSTANT READER – The reason you received no reply is that your signature renders you practically anonymous. We have dozens of 'Constant Readers' writing by every post, and it would be impossible to distinguish them. Put your initials, put anything you like, but pray do not retain the 'Constant Reader.'

– oOo –

A L D I B O R O N T I P H O - SCOPHORNIA – Hooray! That is an improvement on 'Constant Reader'.

– oOo –

ANTINONTONTHOLAGOS – We pity our printer if you often use such signatures as the above ...

– oOo –

SAMOHTSGNINNEJDEER – We admire your brevity, but not your clearness. What do you mean?

– oOo –

ARABI PASHA – How much better it would be if you were to write only under initials, instead of selecting the name of some notorious character! There is nothing novel or praiseworthy about such

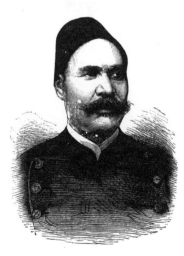

an idea. Every day brings us at least half a dozen letters with the same silly signature. 'Arabi Pasha' is almost as great a nuisance as the 'Constant Reader'.

– o O o –

T. P. (Musselburgh) writes to ask why, in publishing our award in the 'Holiday Letter' competition, we made no reference to *his* letter! He adds, 'I tried for a prize, and sent my letter to you, and am annoyed at not getting an answer to it.' He further asks us to 'fully explain' the meaning of this! If T. P. used only as much intelligence in preparing his MS. as in writing this letter, he ought to have little difficulty in guessing for himself the reason for his name not being mentioned.

– o O o –

You have probably been crowded out. The number of letters you write makes no difference, as our correspondents are too numerous for us to recognise the hand-writing.

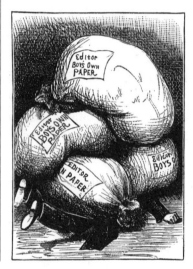

===✕===

Chapter 2

'WHATEVER IS OF INTEREST TO OUR BOYS'

The thirst for knowledge

T HE Latin motto on the front cover of every BOY'S OWN PAPER, *Quidquid agunt pueri nostri farrago libelli,* was usually translated as 'a little book about whatever is of interest to our boys'. One schoolmaster sent in some alternative translations supplied by his class:

> Our boys go anywhere waging warfare.
> Whoever of our boys derive good or bad from these books.
> Our boys do anything to break rules.
> Our boys can drive anything.

The B.O.P.'s idea of what was of interest was eclectic, liberal and, for its time, advanced. As an avowedly Christian publication it nevertheless recognised the merits of the work of Charles Darwin, whose theory of evolution by natural selection was seen by some Christians as a direct attack on their beliefs:

> MEN WHO ARE TALKED ABOUT:– ...Without adopting the Darwinian theory of "evolution," or the development of all crea-tures, man included, from lower forms of life, we cannot but admire the author's shrewd powers of observation and patient industry. His latest work, published not long before his death, on Earthworms, could hardly fail to interest any intelligent boy, and might be read with advantage by all ...

Other areas of science and technology, particularly as they were affecting daily life, also appeared in the B.O.P.'s columns. The telegraph, for example, which was covered in technical articles, was also described from the point of view of a post office telegraphist, who took delight in making fun of people's unfamiliarity with the process of sending a telegram:

> The extraordinary ignorance of everything relating to the telegraph which (and I am speaking from experience) seems to prevail among the great bulk of our population is really astonishing. Of course amongst the lower or working classes this is especially apparent, and many, many hearty laughs do we clerks have behind the scenes... Some customers will present themselves, trembling and nervous, totally unable to collect themselves and write out a clear, concise and distinct message; then is the time for the clerk to exercise calmness, tact and common sense. Other customers, maybe, are anxious to wrangle and dispute about the counting of words and signs; then is patience required, aye, and not unfrequently more patience, I fear, than many of us possess.
>
> I shall not soon forget the amusement afforded at my office one day when a young woman, who was unable to write, presented herself and asked me to pen a message for her. On inquiring the nature of her communication, she replied that she merely wished to let her sister known what time to meet her at — railway station; and then proceeded to dictate a long rigmarole, commencing:
>
> 'My dear sister, I hope to be able...' etc., etc. The message, when she finished, would have cost over two shillings, whereat she was greatly astonished, and "thought it was only sixpence to send a telegram!" After considerable persuasion she allowed it to be cut down by twenty-seven words, but would not on any account hear of leaving out the affectionate parts. All that was needed could have been condensed into a message of twelve words.

...I used to wonder why some people took so much care [to write out carefully] but the cat was let out of the bag by an individual exhorting one of my fellow-assistants to 'mind it was kept clean!' They think that by some occult process the paper is spirited along the wire to its destination; in fact, I was plainly asked one day by an individual who was really old enough to know better, 'How do you fix the paper on the wire?' in all seriousness! ...

As often happens with new technology, people are not always able to foresee the consequences. A regular B.O.P. writer, Arthur Stradling, was convinced that the inventions of the Victorian age would lead to the quick demise of several other technologies, which are actually still with us:

This is certainly an age of marvellous inventions. It is not simply that machines are brought out to do *more* than has been done previously, but discoveries are made and natural laws applied to enable us to accomplish that which has never been effected before in any degree. Not simply that engines are built which run more miles within the hour, cranes which lift heavier weights, and telescopes which pierce further into the depths of the heavens, but that our own voices can be heard half-way across the kingdom, and may be packed up and sent by post more easily than a written letter. And it really seems to have come upon us all at once. Most of you can remember, if not the introduction of the electric light into our streets, at any rate the coming into general use of the telephone; and you will all be able to speak of the first perfect phonograph, the first electric steamer, railway, and tramcar, and the building of the Eiffel Tower, the loftiest structure on the earth. The first time I saw the streets lighted by electricity was in the City of Mexico, and I first spoke through the telephone at Pernambuco, from the offices of my friend, Mr. Elliott, the constructing engineer of the Great Western Railway of Brazil, to his son's hut along the line through the forest.

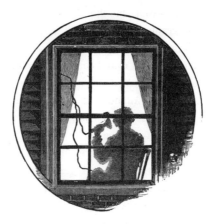

It is really fortunate that some of these inventions do not do quite all they threaten to do at first, or the world would be turned upside down. The telephone was going to leave us no secrets at all: every word we spoke would be heard by our neighbours, and even by those afar off, by simply putting a wire through a keyhole. But we know now that even where the proper instrument is fitted and connected to a room, general conversation is by no means audible to those at the other end, and that we must speak deliberately over the apparatus to be heard at all. So it is rather to be hoped that the phonograph, the queer machine which records what is said to it on thin sheets of tinfoil, and actually talks it back to us in the same voice when required – one hopes, I say, that this phonograph will *not* carry out everything that its inventor promises. Somebody said the other day that it will be of no use to learn writing any longer, as this instrument will quite take the place of the pen. You speak into it instead of writing a letter, take out the dotted strip of foil and send it to your friend in Australia or New York, and he puts it into his phonograph, and your own voice delivers your message to him. And it is foretold, too, that we shall have no more news-papers, magazines, or printed books (so I suppose we may give up learning to read as well), but that the news will be talked out to us by the phonograph on the breakfast-table, speeches will be reported not only in the words but in the accents of the speakers, and at night we shall all sit round comfortably and listen while our favourite author is turned on. But I imagine it will stop somewhere short of this. Anyhow, they won't be able to phonograph the BOY'S OWN PAPER – for you can't talk pictures.

There is another appliance now which reproduces your very handwriting, or a drawing if you like. You use a pencil to which a wire is attached, and at the other end, miles away, another pencil writes and draws in exact imitation. And it is thought possible that light will eventually be conveyed in like manner, and that we shall be able to see scenes at a distance through the medium of a wire.

(Now that really is fantastical ...)

But Stradling was more pessimistic about the promise of another new invention, an early version of the typewriter:

Authors, I think, do not use the type-writer much yet. You do not *see* what you are writing, and cannot readily refer a line or two back, and that must be awkward to any but a very rapid and accurate writer, and one who has an abundance of words at his command, so that he is in no danger of using the same twice in a short space. Besides, to break in upon established custom often interferes with the flow of ideas. Years ago, when I was living abroad and wrote a good deal more than I do now, someone gave me one of those stylographic pens – a sort of pencil-case which was filled with ink, and did not want replenishing for days[i.e. a fountain pen]. It acted perfectly. They were expensive things, and, if I am not mistaken, cost then fifteen shillings apiece. But I could not write with it! – could not get on without that momentary interval occupied in the passage of the hand to the inkstand.

You could find facts about science, history, geography, art, and the world in general in issues of the B.O.P. Single paragraphs like the following, as well as long articles:

Great Men's Hobbies

The grave philosophic Socrates, during his leisure hours, took pleasure in dancing. Luther delighted in the flute, and this used to soothe his excited feelings... Milton delighted in playing the organ... Gainsborough, the painter, was a performer on the violin. Byron's delight was in flowers; he was also fond of animals and in his youth he made a friend of a bear. Goethe rarely passed a day without bringing out from the chimney corner a live snake, which he kept there and caressed. Tiberius, the Roman, made companion of a serpent. Augustus was fond of a parrot, but still more so of a quail, the loss of which made him as mad as if he had lost a battle. Honorius was so grieved at the loss of a hen that he would have given Rome itself to bring it back. Louis XI, when ill, only found pleasure in an exhibition of dancing pigs, oddly dressed up... Rembrandt loved nothing so much as his monkey... Pelisson, confined in the Bastille, made a friend of a spider, which he tamed. The Marquis de Montespan amused himself with mice when occupying the gilded apartments at Versailles.

A similar eclecticism was reflected in the general knowledge queries sent in by readers, sometimes, it appears, just for the sake of testing the knowledge of 'the Editor'. Many boys submitted multiple questions, and got multiple answers:

INQUIRER NO. 1. – asks us to answer no less than eighteen questions, and to recommend him the best books for studying a whole page of diversified subjects, ranging from astronomy, oil-painting, and universal history, down to kitchen gardening for a cottager. We have no space. Some friend should advise him.

J.C. RENOUF – What feeds a sheep will feed a goat. Whiting or hard fine chalk. Camphorated chalk. Bathing after sunset may be dangerous to some constitutions. Your sister should leave her eyebrows alone.

– oOo –

From your letter we should infer a very different opinion of you than you say your friends do. We fail to see why 'Blacks' should put Singapore on the map of Europe. If you look at the map of Asia you will probably find that he has put it in the proper place at the South of the Malayan Peninsula. We would rather not have your 'writings' on silkworms. The length of an elephant's tail is not invariable. Tusks have been met with weighing three hundred and fifty pounds. We never heard of 'verdy-greece' on the teeth, but suppose it would brush off; and we have no space to answer all your inquiries.

– oOo –

L.J.M., AND A HOST OF OTHERS – Ingrowing toenails were treated in No. 101; the Australian Cricketers were in No. 97; the national arms in No. 107, and the plate in the February part; the limelight query in No. 122; the pigeon articles, fourteen in all, commenced in No. 109; perch-fishing in No. 80; tench-fishing in No. 83; and the kite-carriage articles in Nos. 93, 94, 95, and 96. All those not answered should get the indexes. That to the last volume is very detailed. Have received your letter. When we have a couple of pages to spare we will answer your thirty-eight queries.

– oOo –

1. Stop the rape. I suppose you mean a canary, though you don't say so. 2. Your sister is right.

– oOo –

1. 'Night closed fast' means that day ended. 2. For words ending in 'dous' – stupendous, tremendous, and so on – look through the dictionary for yourself. 3. Almost any music seller could supply you with the songs. 4. Try Russian corn solvent, which principally consists of hemp. 5. There is a Horseshoe Lake in California. 6. Better buy your ink ready-made. There are ink-powders sold for export which may be useful to you. 7. Indian clubs for a boy of sixteen should

weigh about eight pounds for each club.

– oOo –

You ask over the average number of questions, but you are American, and we readily forgive you. 1. Eighteen pence a dozen eggs (from home farm). 2. From 1s. 6d. to 2s. 3. From 2s. 6d. to 3s. 6d. 4. Rent of such a house as you name would be about £28, with taxes; and count the land at £3 an acre. The farther from a station the cheaper, but say a mile. 4[*sic*]. Anywhere near or within cheap access to a city such as London, Edinburgh, Glasgow, Manchester, etc. 5. The best poultry book out is Wright's, published by Cassell and Co.

– oOo –

Our correspondents would oblige by using short *noms de plume,* as our space is very valuable. 1. Bird no use. 2. No one can prevent you egg-collecting, but you can be summoned for trespass. 3. We do not think so. 4. No, an air-pistol is not firearms. 5. With a knife.

– oOo –

1. No man's debts are paid by his staying away from a town, and no man with any sense of honour would think of doing such a thing. 2. The name of her Majesty was the same after her marriage as it was before, as the slightest knowledge of history would have told you. 3. We really cannot decide questions as to the amount of crèpe you should wear for your grandmother.

– oOo –

1. The tar will dry in time no matter how sticky it may be. 2. We are going to have an article on bowling in the good time coming. 3. Keep the dog off any other food for a time. 4. We have had articles on swimming, the best ever published. [*The phrase 'a good time coming' was used several times by the Editor and is taken from a popular song by Charles Mackay.*]

– oOo –

1. To clear cork of insects the best way is to bake it. 2. For photographs of engines you must apply to the locomotive superintendent.

– oOo –

Yes. No. North Pole. Moreton Bay. Perhaps. Thanks. Try boiled oil. Half-a-crown. Queen Emma.

Buckingham Palace. Black your boots. We have answered all the Constant Readers together this batch, and you must sort out your answers for yourselves. Why will you use a signature that is practically anonymous?

– oOo –

1. 'What is the proper way of ending a hammock?' See our articles. 2. 'Was George Eliott a man or a woman?' As you spell it, George Eliott was a man; but George Eliot the novelist was a lady – Mary Ann Evans, Mrs. G.H. Lewes, afterwards Mrs. Crosse – born in 1820, died in 1881. 3. 'How can I become a good cricketer?' By steady, intelligent practice, and carefully reading our articles by Dr. W.G. Grace. 4. 'It being my intention to become Prime Minister, would you kindly state the way I am to set about it?' Really! We cannot say. We have no articles on this subject, and must give it up. The responsibility of advising you would be too great.

– oOo –

1. We have really no means of knowing if there is any chance of your getting rich. 2. Armed to the teeth means armed as much as it is possible to be armed – in other words, armed even to the teeth, which are generally supposed to need no arming. 3. We have no room for amateur puzzles.

– oOo –

1. The fee at Stationers' Hall is five shillings. 2. In all cases the person who gets possession of the property takes over the liabilities to which the property was subject before it came to him, unless there is an express provision to the contrary. It does not matter whether the survivor be a poor widow or a millionaire. 3. You have probably got some insect in your room. It may be a leaf or something blowing against the window-pane. Under any circumstances it is not a ghost, and you can easily clear it up for yourself if you try.

– oOo –

FRENCH POODLE! 1. It is not considered an 'unhelthy sine' for you to have a 'dry noze.' 2. The words you select for your 'charads for a charitible purpuse' had better be extremely simple, as you may find a leetle difficulty in spelling them. 3. We cannot recommend a 'preperation' to blacken your 'caroty' hair, but there are many reasons why you should leave it alone. MARQUIS OF CARABBAS (!) We are unable to suggest a remedy for the 'poor old cat which has got the gout very bad on its off-side foreleg.' 4. The 'toffe' which 'always goes to squash' is evidently not made properly. [*A recipe follows.*] 5. Lear was not 'a fabulous monster,' but a legendary King of Britain; and the story is told about Ina, King of the West Saxons. Percy's 'Reliques' has a ballad on the subject. Geoffrey of Monmouth gives it in his Chronicles; Holinshed copied it from these, and Spenser introduces it in the 'Faery Queene'. The less said about these specimens of spelling and writing the better.

– oOo –

1. The helmet in 'Sigurd' is of the usual ancient Norse form. 2. We see no difficulty in eating seventeen slices of bread-and-butter – it all depends on their dimensions!

– oOo –

1. In the catechism M stands for double N, the symbol for Names, and N stands for name. In the marriage service M stands for Maritus the bridegroom, and N for Nupta the bride. M may stand for Mary, the patron saint of girls; and N for Nicholas, the patron saint of boys; but this is not generally admitted. 2. The inventor of the modern bicycle was either James Starley, of Coventry, or the hundreds who preceded him. 3. Eton claims to be the public school of most ancient special foundation, but the Abbey and Cathedral schools have a longer descent. 4. Leave the bird alone.

– oOo –

1. Yes, Rider Haggard is alive, and likely to be so for some time. 2. Paint your chilblains twice a day with opodeldoc. What is the connection between Rider Haggard and chilblains?

– oOo –

1. A newly-married man is not called a Benedict, but a Benedick, and the reason you will discover on reading Shakespeare's 'Much Ado about Nothing.' Spinster is from the spinning which was formerly the work of the unmarried girls. 2. Roundheads were so

called from their wearing their hair cut short, as we wear it now. 3. We do not see stars in the daylight because of the diffused light of the sun; but if you look up a tall chimney that light is shut out, and you see the stars. [*A rare example of an erroneous answer – you can't see the stars in the daytime from the bottom of a chimney.*] 4. Why are there so many questions from Harrogate by one delivery? Why do you write on postcards? Why this triplet fashion?

– o O o –

1. For small quantities of circulars and so forth. 2. Walk on. 3. Not unless you have been introduced. 4. No. 5. On the right hand. 6. Allowable. Why not buy a book? You can get one for a shilling. 7. Wherever you like, and whichever you please.

There was always a proportion of queries about topics which today we would consider 'fringe'. On the whole the Editor showed a healthy scepticism in an age when spiritualism was rampant and irrational beliefs could still held by many intelligent people. The *Correspondence* columns also displayed a compendious general knowledge, in the days when, if you didn't know an answer, you would have to spend a considerable amount of time in a well-stocked library to find it:

A pure delusion, akin to witchcraft and other superstitions. Nothing was ever found in the earth by means of a divining-rod but what had already been previously discovered on the quiet at the indicated spot. It is simply an imposture practised on fools, and foolishly published by a foolish reporter. You would find a shilling book of geology to be much more effective in enabling you to discover the whereabouts of minerals and springs than a whole cartload of hazel switches.

– o O o –

There is no such science, and such a book would be an imposture. You can no more tell our character from our handwriting than you can tell it from our type.

– o O o –

We said thunderbolts have no existence, and we meant it. The slightest knowledge of electricity will tell you why. The fact of 'a statement somewhere' that three successive Kings of Ireland were killed by thunderbolts does not prove the existence of thunderbolts, or even the existence of the kings!

– oOo –

You need not alarm yourself, the report was circulated in error. Mr. Proctor, in his own paper, 'Knowledge,' gave an article on the 17th February last, in which he denies having said that the world was coming to an end at any fixed date, by any means, cometary or otherwise. A greater than he has told us that 'the time and season knoweth no man.'

– oOo –

The answer is simply that a watch WILL go on a marble mantelpiece unless there is something the matter with the watch which would prevent its going in the same position on anything else ...

– oOo –

When you get more enlarged notions of the immensity of space, your fear and curiosity will vanish, and comets, however large or near, will cease to trouble you. Our forefathers used to think that comets portended most dreadful things; but then their ideas of the relative importance of our small planet in the scheme of the universe were somewhat exaggerated. The mermaids had as much existence at the City griffin. The specimen exhibited at the Aquarium was a manatee, and the manatee is the animal which is the basis of the mermaid legend.

– oOo –

As you have only 'just heard' of the zodiac, it is rather difficult to explain its meaning to you clearly.

– oOo –

There are such things as electric engines used for organ blowing, but we know nothing about their price. Apply at the Albert Hall. Of course they do not explode; why should they?

– oOo –

The last words of Anaxagoras were, 'Give the lads a holiday.'

– oOo –

1. Music is always sold at half the price named on it because it is marked at double the price it is intended to sell it at, and all the profits on its sale and production are calculated on its so-called half-price.

– o O o –

A country dance is not necessarily of country origin. The word is a corruption of the French 'contre danse' – so called from the partners facing each other.

– o O o –

Somewhat obvious. A claptrap sentence is a sentence so made and uttered as to afford a trap for an approving clap. A claptrap speech is simply a trap for clapping without any regard to honesty or reason.

– o O o –

We never heard of the tournament of Acre. We are not prepared to discuss in these columns whether Oliver Cromwell was justified in 'murdering Charles I' – in fact, it is the first time we hear that he did so; and we quite agree with you that if we were to insert 'selections from Sir Walter Scott, Shakespeare, and Lord Macaulay, the poetry would be better than it now is.' Your

chronology is rather shaky. Vespasian was not born till A.D. 9. A genuine Roman coin, bearing the date B.C. 80, is indeed a rarity. If it were not for the extraordinary date it would be worth about a shilling.

– o O o –

The depth of ignorance on the part of your friends that your letter reveals is absolutely appalling. Do they imagine that ships going to America sail uphill? The reason the voyage from New York to Queenstown takes less time than that from Queenstown to New York is that the prevailing winds and set of the currents are in an easterly direction – a direction due to the revolution of the earth on its axis and the difference of temperature between the equator and the poles.

– o O o –

We are unable to remember a book 'that gives an insight into the cutting-out of trousers,' but would suggest that an old pair taken to pieces would answer every purpose. In the event of one pair only being available, a modification of the Highland costume might be adopted for the nonce.

– o O o –

It is quite true. By the twitchings of the man's muscles, Dr. Hughes Bennet discovered that a tumour of limited dimensions was ensconced at a particular point on the ascending frontal convolution on the right side of the brain, and so he opened the patient's skull, and exactly at the spot indicated a tumour about the size of a walnut was found. The tumour was removed, and the patient recovered.

– o O o –

Richard I was the first to use 'Dieu et Mon Droit.' We confess it had not occurred to us before, but it certainly does seem absurd that we have not yet had the sense to adopt a national motto in our own tongue. However, there's a good time coming, you know.

– o O o –

We do not know what you mean by a square acre, as we have never yet heard of an acre that was not square. The acreage of England and Wales is 37,239,351.

– o O o –

There is no law compelling carriages to carry lighted lamps at night, but there ought to be. Such things are left to by-laws, which vary in different districts, and are never held in much respect.

– o O o –

If the earth's atmosphere were removed the sun would still illuminate a hemisphere – but there would be no one here to see it.

– o O o –

Oil copies of old masters, particularly in the case of sacred subjects are of very little value; and your picture is probably worth only the price of the frame.

– o O o –

John Gibson, the sculptor, measured the Queen for a statue, and according to him she was then exactly five feet high. What her height is now we do not know, but it is probably less than that.

– o O o –

No one has ever seen the fiery state in the centre of the earth. There is little reason for supposing it exists, and there are many reasons why it should not exist – in fact, the theory is being slowly given up. We do not know what will be the doom of the earth, nor do we know how long the sun will last. You should be far better employed in preparing for your own death than in making arrangements for the collapse of the universe.

– oOo –

It is not worth while to say anything about your discovery. You simply support the well-known fact that stopping trains run faster from station to station than expresses do. Many other instances than the one you name could be given. The time is saved by not stopping at the station. On no line is there an express running on short distances faster than a stopping train.

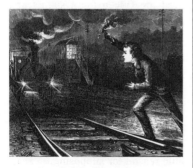

– oOo –

The star that appeared a few months ago, and caused you so much perturbation, is simply the planet Venus, which can be seen now if you will only take the trouble to look for it, and no more requires 'explaining' than does the sun. There was nothing wonderful about the affair except the ignorance which made a wonder of the most familiar star in the sky. [*Another rare lapse – surely the Editor knows that Venus is not a star?*]

– oOo –

SARDINES – There is no mystery in the matter. The same fish has two names – when it is young it is called sardine, when it is full grown it is called pilchard; in fact the sardine is simply the young of the pilchard. Any modern encyclopaedia or book on fishes will tell you this. 'Pilchards dressed like sardines' is much as if you were to say 'Men dressed as boys!'

– oOo –

Look at the almanac. If the almanac does not give the time of high water it may give the moon's age. If it gives the moon's age remember the old rhyme:

'Four times the moon's age if by
   five you divide,
Gives the hour of her southing;
   add two for the tide'

– oOo –

Is it possible to have two stepmothers? We suppose it is, though we never thought about it before. How was it with Henry VIII's children? How many stepmothers had Elizabeth? There's a little historical exercise for you.

– o O o –

There is no doubt about it. The statement must have been copied from some older book. It is now admitted that whitebait are young herrings. As soon as the anatomy was studied all ground for difference was removed.

– o O o –

We do not know where Suva is – but, then, we are not under examination. You may depend upon it there is a town of that name in the United States. Every name in geography is duplicated there. [*One year later, in another answer, the Editor had done his research.*]

– o O o –

Suva is one of the Fiji Islands.

– o O o –

A CORRESPONDENT – is desirous of knowing if the following is true. Is it possible for a doubt to exist on the subject? Wonderful things happen at the North Pole! 'I have heard that when sailors are at the North Pole it freezes so hard that when the captain gives them an order they have to pick up the frozen words and put them in a frying-pan for twenty minutes to thaw them; and when they want any butter they have to chip it off with a hammer and a chisel!' He has another question as to experiences round Cape Horn – but we refrain.

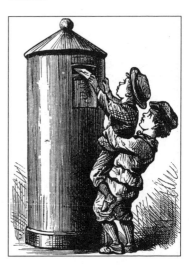

=✗=

HISTORY AND MYTH

DEATHS

Charles VIII was the king that died from hitting his head against a doorpost; Frederick Lewis, Prince of Wales, died from a blow of a cricket-ball. Some of the Greeks are reported to have had strange deaths. Anacreon was choked with a grape-stone; Aeschylus was knocked on the head by a tortoise dropped from the claws of an eagle; Agathocles swallowed his toothpick; and Zeuxis laughed himself to death at the sight of one of his own pictures. Zeuxis was not a comic artist.

COAL

Coals were known to the Britons before the arrival of the Romans. The Romans knew nothing of coals till they came to this country. They had no name for them in their language.

ARGUS

Argus was the son of Arestor. He was very strong and killed a wild bull, and the Echidna, which was not the duck-mole, but half a snake and half a woman. He had a hundred eyes and only two went to sleep at a time, and altogether was such a very remarkable individual that he has now given his name to a bicycle club.

GELERT

The story of Gelert is told in the Gesta Romanorum as having occurred to Folliculus, who, on his repentance, makes a pilgrimage to the Holy Land. In the Pantschatantra the hero is Devasaman, the dog being an ichneumon. In Nasr Allah's Arabic version the dog becomes a weasel. In the Mongolian Uligerun the dog is a polecat.

=✗=

In the Persian Hitopadesa the dog is an otter; and in the Sindibadnameh it is a cat. There is a Hebrew version in which the dog is a dog, as in Wales. The resemblances do not disprove the fact that the incident might have happened to Llywelin.

KNIGHT

There were many ceremonies to be gone through before a young man was knighted. It is only in these later days that the mere accolade suffices. The candidate had to fast, and watch his armour in the dark church, doing penance and taking the sacrament, and undergoing a regular process of initiation. Previous to their coronation our old kings had to go through a similar ordeal.

ENGLISH USURPERS

In such a mere matter of opinion you cannot say an examiner was wrong. You should have taken the text-book recommended for the examination, and followed what it says on the subject. You can make out at least eleven usurpers of the English throne. William Rufus 'usurped' in place of Robert; Henry I in place of Robert; Stephen in place of Matilda; John in place of Arthur; Henry IV in place of Edmund Mortimer; Henry V in place of Edmund Mortimer; Henry VI in place of Richard of York; Richard III in place of Edward V; Henry VII in place of Edward Earl of Warwick; William III in place of James II; and George I in place of the Old Pretender. Anne, too, could be called a usurper. Even Mary and Elizabeth could be looked upon as usurpers. But where are you to stop? On the other hand, it is possible to show that none of these were usurpers – not even Stephen – for they all reigned by the wish of the people, and the right of election was never parted with. Usurpations before the Conquest are never thought worthy of mention; and yet look at the number of sons that had to make room for their uncles!

BRAVE MOHAMMEDANS

Jaafar was killed at the battle of Muta, the first fight in which the valour of the Moslems was tried against a foreign enemy. Zeid, the slave of Mahomet, who was freed on his conversion, was the bearer of the sacred banner, Jaafar and Abdallah being ordered to succeed him should he be killed. The struggle was most obstinate, and Zeid fell fighting desperately in the very front rank. Jaafar seized the banner, but lost his right hand. He shifted the standard to his left; the left was severed from his body, and then he embraced the flag with his bleeding stumps till he was transfixed to the ground with fifty honourable wounds. 'Advance!' cried Abdallah, who stepped into the vacant place – 'advance with confidence; either victory or paradise is our own.' The lance of a Roman decided the alternative, but Caled seized the standard as it fell. Nine swords were broken in his hand, but he fought on grimly and relentlessly, and his valour withstood and repulsed the superior numbers of the 'Christians.' It is a great mistake to speak slightingly of the bravery of the founders of Mohammedanism. Their motives are another thing.

CATO STREET

The Cato Street conspiracy was originated by Arthur Thistlewood, Ings (a butcher), Tidd (a shoemaker), Brunt (a shoemaker), and Davidson (a negro). The object was to murder the Ministers when they were at dinner at Lord Harrowby's on the 23rd of February, to set fire to London in different places at once, to seize the Bank and Mansion House, and proclaim a provisional Government. A man named Edwards joined it for the purpose of giving information, so that the authorities were aware of all that was going on. 'Cato Street' has had its name altered to Little Bryanston Street, near Edgware Road.

THUMBS DOWN

A correspondent writes: 'I feel sure that you will excuse me for pointing out that in your issue of January 28 your illustrator of M. Gerome's picture, 'Doomed to Die,' has fallen into the error of which the artist has also been guilty. He says, 'the people give the well-known fatal signal by turning down their thumbs.' Now, sir, a moment's reflection will, I am sure, convince you that this statement is misleading, and likely to give your youthful readers a wrong impression of the actual custom. To press down the thumb (premere) was a sign of approbation at play, vide Pliny, xxviii. 2. 5, *'Pollices, cum faveamus, premere etiam proverbio jubemur*,' see also Horace, (*'Fautor utroque tuum laudabit pollice ludum'*), Epist. i. 18. 66, where the custom is fully explained in Dr. Maclean's edition of the poet. On the other hand, the sign of disapprobation (which M. Gerome of course intended to represent) was the extension of the thumb. This is set beyond doubt by Juvenal, iii. 36, *'Verso pollice vulgi quemlibet occidunt populariter.'* Had your magazine been intended for general reading merely such a slip would not have been of much moment, but in the case of a publication of such authority as the BOY'S OWN PAPER it seems to me that the consequences may be serious.'

TALL MEN

There have been many recorded instances. Joseph Brice (Anak) was 7ft. 8in. high; Edward Bamford, 7ft. 4in.; Captain Bates, 7ft. 11½ in.; Henry Blacker, 7ft. 4in.; Bradley (whose hand is at the College of Surgeons), 7ft. 8in.; John Busby, 7ft. 9in.; Chang, 8ft. 2in.; Charles the Great, nearly 8ft.; Patrick Cotter, 8ft. 7½in.; Joachim Eleizegue, 7ft. 10in.; William Evans (Charles I's porter), 8ft.; Francis Sheridan, 7ft. 8in.; Louis Frenz, 7ft. 4in.; Alice Gordon, 7ft.; Robert Hale, 7ft. 6in.; Harold Hardrada, 7ft. 10in.;

Lovshkin (Russian drum-major – $1/2$ maximus!), 8ft. 5in.; James McDonald, 7ft. 6in.; Samuel McDonald (Prince of Wales's footman), 6ft. 10in.; Cornelius Magrath (educated by Bishop Berkeley, who yet doubted the existence of matter!), 7ft. 8in.; Marian, now in London, 8ft. 2in.; Maximinius, the Roman emperor, 8ft. 6in.; Edmund Mellon, 7ft. 6in.; John Middleton, 9ft. 3in.; Charles O'Brien (whose skeleton is in Lincoln's Inn Fields), 8ft. 4in.; Heinrich Osen (weighed $37^{1}/2$ stone!), 7ft. 6in.; Porus (Alexander's friend), 7ft. 6in.; Riechart, 8ft. 3in.; and ever so many more. King Frederick William of Prussia (Frederick the Great's father) had a whole regiment of giants, all over 7ft high.

FEASTS

The moveable feasts of the year depend upon Easter, and Easter depends, not upon the movements of any of the heavenly bodies, but of an imaginary new moon, specially invented to prevent the Jewish Passover at any time clashing with the Christian Feast, and so designed that it always follows the real new moon by two or three days. Notwithstanding the intention, Easter and Passover have occasionally coincided, and will do so again. We keep Easter in the mode of the Western Churches, but the Eastern Churches adhere to the Jewish Calendar. At the Council of the Nicaea in 325 this was the question discussed, and the schism became permanent. Britain, having been converted to Christianity under the Empire by the Roman legionaries, etc., adhered to the older fashion in keeping Easter, and hence the British Church was denounced as unorthodox by Augustine when he arrived here on his mission to the English. When the Gregorian Calendar was being introduced it was proposed to make Easter a fixed and not a moveable feast, but the design had to be abandoned owing to the opposition of those who considered that the ecclesiastical moon, and the moveability of the date, had some mystical significance. Easter can never come before the 23rd of March or after the 25th of April.

HELPFUL SAINTS

What does St. Christopher do? Well, he protects you from unpleasant dreams, rescues you from flood, puts out your house when on fire, supports you during an earthquake, and, like a freely-advertised night-light, is the 'burglars' horror' in defying robbery. If you have got the toothache, appeal to St. Blaise, who also makes a speciality of the quinsy and pleuro-pneumonia. If you have the ague, try St. Pernel, or St. Petronella; if neuralgia, try St. Apollonia; if you have bad eyes, try St. Clare – or spectacles; if you have a bad boil, inform St. Rooke; if you have the colic, St. Erasmus is the authority; if the gout, you should go to St. Wolfgang; if the leprosy, St. Lazarus; if the smallpox, St. Martin of Tours. Those who want riches should apply to St. Anne and St. Vincent; those who have lost their umbrellas should go to St. Ethelbert or St. Elian, – or Scotland Yard. There were even saints credited with special powers as flea and beetle exterminators, such as St. Gertrude and St. Huldrick. But, enough; to quote the absurdities of saint-worship is but slaying the slain. In an antiquarian sense, however, the facts are interesting. There is a long list of saints for diseases, patron saints of places, and patron saints of trades and professions, in Brewer's *Readers' Handbook.*

ROYAL COCK CROWER

There was an officer of the royal household with the title of the 'King's Cock Crower.' The office, however, was abolished in the reign of George I. The crowing gentleman's last appearance was during a supper given by George II, then Prince of Wales. The door opened, and in came an aristocratic individual in a gorgeous costume, announcing himself as 'Cockadoodleoo! It's ten o'clock! Ten o'clock! Cockadoodleooodleooodleoo!' The Prince was angry, thinking the affair was a Jacobite insult; but on the facts being explained to him he put up his sword, and the King's Cockcrowership was soon afterwards abolished.

PEOPLE

ADMIRABLE CRICHTON

James Crichton, the 'Admirable Crichton,' was a Scotch scholar of encyclopaedic attainments, who was born in 1560, and died when he was only twenty-three. He was one of the handsomest athletes of his time, a practised linguist, and astonished all Italy by his off-hand discourses on theology, philosophy, and such like themes. He was tutor to the son of the Duke of Mantua, and one night was attacked in the streets by a band of masked men. He beat them off, and recognised one of them as his pupil. To him he at once offered his sword, and the Italian took it, and ran him through with it.

LADY GODIVA

The legend is that Leofric, Earl of Mercia, in 1040 levied a tax on his people at Coventry, and that his wife Godiva begged him to abolish it. To get rid of her importunity, he promised to do so if she would ride nude through the town; and this, trusting to her abundant hair for concealment, she did. The inhabitants of the town kept indoors at the time, but a certain tailor named Thomas peeped at the lady as she passed. The whole thing is a fiction of comparatively recent date. Leofric, the great and good Earl of Mercia, was the very last man to have said such a thing, and his wife Godgifu the very last woman who would have done it. Leofric and Godgifu were always much attached to each other; they did many good deeds and built many churches, among them the minster of Coventry, which afterwards became the cathedral church, and was pulled down in the time of Henry VIII. If there had been a Thomas in Coventry in those days he would have been some wretched foreigner, for then and for some time afterwards Englishmen did not use Scriptural names.

NOMS DE PLUME

Artemus Ward is the assumed name of Charles F. Browne; Aunt Fanny of Mrs. F.D. Gage; Barry Gray of Robert B. Coffin; Hosea Biglow of James Russell Lowell; Josh Billings of Henry W. Shaw; Bob Short of A.B. Longstreet; Hans Breitmann of C.G. Leland; Vandyke Brown of W.P. Brannan; Ned Buntline of E.Z. Judson; Christopher Caustic of T.G. Fessenden; Laura Caxton of Lizzie B. Comries; Geoffrey Crayon of Washington Irving; Porte Crayon of D.P. Strother; Shirley Dare of Susan Dunning; Q.K. Philander Doesticks of M.N. Thompson; Dunn Brown of Samuel Fiske; Edmund Kirke of J.R. Gilmore; Elizabeth Wetherell of Susan Warner; Ethan Spike of M.F. Whittier; Fanny Fern of Sarah Parton; Fanny Fielding of Mary Upshur; Fanny Forester of Emily Judson; Fat Contributor of A.M. Griswold; Alfred Armitage of William Murray Graydon; Florence Leigh of Anna T. Wilbur; Tom Folio of J.E. Babson; Francis Oldys of George Chalmers; Frank Forrester of W.H. Herbert; Howard Glyndon of Laura Reddon; Grace Greenwood of Sarah Lippincott; Major Jack Downing of Seba Smith; Orpheus C. Kerr of R.H. Newell; Mark Twain of Samuel L. Clemens; J.K. Marvell of Donald Mitchell; Petroleum V. Nasby of David R. Locke; Oliver Optic of W.T. Adams; Mrs. Partington of B.P. Shillaber; Peter Schlemihl of George Wood; Poor Richard of Benjamin Franklin; Sam Slick of T.C. Haliburton; Timothy Titcomb of J.G. Holland.

CHRISTIANITY

It is not really known who first preached the Gospel in Britain. St. Alban is said to have been the first martyr, in 304. When Christianity became the established church of the Roman Empire, Britain, like the rest of the empire, grew nominally Christian – the legions, in fact, were missionary centres. In Roman times there were three archbishoprics here – London, York, and Caerleon – and these lasted till the English conquest. When the pagan Saxons came the Christian Romano-Britons were driven to the fastnesses of the west, and the country was pagan again for one hundred and fifty years. When Augustine arrived, however, he found Ethelbert's Christian queen worshipping at St. Martin's Canterbury, under Bishop Luidhard. Augustine was *not* the great Augustine, and he did *not* convert the Britons.

PHYSICAL FACTS

The average height of Englishmen is 5ft. 7½ in.The height depends a good deal on social condition and nurture. Men who work with their heads are taller than those who work with their hands; there are exceptions, of course, but 'the big brain in the little body' theory is not borne out by statistics. The criminal classes are the shortest in stature, the average being 5ft. 5½in. The professional classes are the tallest in stature, the average being 5ft. 9in. The average height of the Yankee and the Britisher is exactly the same; and the average height of the English-speaking races is more than two inches greater than that of the rest of the world.

Your height is greatest in the morning. As a rule the inhabitants of towns are taller than those that dwell in the country. At nineteen the boy and girl are the same height as they will be in old age. The maximum weight is reached in the fortieth year.

There are many well-authenticated instances of men and women living for more than a hundred years. Attila, the great King of the Huns, who overran Europe, but who was at last driven back over the Rhine, died at the age of 124. Margaret Patten died at the age of 137; the Countess of Desmond attained 145; Thomas Parr died at 152; and Peter Torton died at 185.

DOCTORS OF THE CHURCH

The Greek Church recognises St. Athanasius, St. Basil, St. Gregory of Nyssa, and St. John Chrysostom; while the Latin Church recognises St. Augustine, St. Jerome, St. Ambrose, and St. Gregory the Great. If you mean the scholastic doctors, the list is a formidable one. As a few examples we may mention Roger Bacon, who was the 'Admirable Doctor' and the 'Wonderful Doctor'; Thomas Aquinas, the 'Angelic Doctor' and the 'Universal Doctor'; Gregory of Rimini, the 'Authentic Doctor'; Jean Ruysbroek, the 'Divine Doctor' and the 'Ecstatic Doctor'; Antonio Andreas, the 'Dulcifluous Doctor'; Peter Aureolus, the 'Eloquent Doctor'; Wycliffe, the 'Evangelical Doctor'; Raymond Lully, the 'Most Enlightened Doctor'; Occam, the 'Invincible Doctor' and the 'Singular Doctor'; Alexander Hales, the 'Irrefragible Doctor'; St. Bernard, the 'Mellifluous Doctor'; Jean de Gerson, the 'Most Christian Doctor'; John Bassol, the 'Most Methodical Doctor'; Aegidius de Colonna, the 'Most Profound Doctor'; Walter Burley, the 'Perspicuous Doctor'; Bradwardine, the 'Profound Doctor'; Anselm of Laon, the 'Scholastic Doctor'; St. Bonaventura, the 'Seraphic Doctor'; Henry Goethals, the 'Solemn Doctor'; Richard Middleton, the 'Solid Doctor'; Duns Scotus, the 'Subtle Doctor'; William Varro, the 'Thorough Doctor'; William de Champeaux, the 'Venerable Doctor'; Aegidius Romanus, the 'Well-founded Doctor'; and Wessel, the 'Wise Doctor'.

LORD PAGET'S AXIOMS

The axioms of Lord Paget of Beaudesert. The complete list, as given in his commonplace book, is:

Flye the courte,
Speke little,
Care less,
Devise nothing,
Never ernest,
In answer cold,
Lerne to spare;
Spend with measure,
Care for home,
Pray often,
Live better,
And dye well.

Paget was a very successful man – but success is not everything!

SLEEPERS

General Pichegru is said to have been satisfied during his campaigns with one hour's sleep out of the twenty-four, Wellington frequently with three hours, Frederick the Great and John Hunter required only four hours, as also did Elliott, Lord Heathfield, who defended Gibraltar. Quin, the actor, was wont to do twenty-four hours at a stretch; and Dr. Reid, the Scotch metaphysician, used to upset all calculations by sleeping straight on for two days! Plants sleep as well as animals.

CABIN BOY TO ADMIRAL

Cock Thorpe is a Norfolk village, close to Burnham Thorpe, where Nelson was born. It consists of three houses, in each of which an admiral was born! The admirals were Sir Christopher Mings, Sir John Narborough, and Sir Cloudesley Shovel, known in naval history as 'the Cockthorpe admirals.' They all began life as cabin-boys.

JOAN OF ARC

You need not trouble about the date on which Joan of Arc was burnt, or who burnt her, for she was not burnt at all. She married a Robert des Armoise, had several children, and died at a good old age in receipt of a comfortable pension for her services against the English. The whole story, like the famous sinking of the Vengeur exploded by Carlyle, is a mere myth. There seems to have been a woman burnt by the French (not the English, who in the old days got the credit of the brutality) in 1431, but M. Vignier, the latest authority, has proved that she was not the Maid of Orleans, as has been for so many years so confidently stated.

THE QUEEN IS A MAN

If the Queen were like another woman and took her husband's name, her surname would be Wettin, for that was Prince Albert's surname, if he had one – which he had not in the usual interpretation of the word. But by law the Queen is a man, and consequently does not take her husband's name, and she is the representative of a family that has always been sufficiently distinguishable without the necessity of having a surname. The royal houses with surnames have been those that have risen from the ranks since surnames came into fashion, such as the Plantagenets, the Tudors, the Stewarts, etc. In short, the Queen has no surname.

PRODIGIES

When Sir William Rowan Hamilton, the Astronomer-Royal for Ireland, was three years old, he could read well and do the first four rules of arithmetic; by the time he was four he had gained a good knowledge of geography; at five he was able to read and translate Latin, Greek, and Hebrew; at eight he had mastered

French and Italian; at nine he had studied Arabic and Sanscrit; at eleven he compiled a Syriac grammar; and at thirteen he could write letters in Persian! The late Professor H. J. S. Smith could read when he was two years old, and before he was twelve had read all Thucydides, Sophocles, Juvenal, Persius, and Sallust, twelve books of Tacitus, several plays of Aeschylus and Euripides, and a considerable amount of Hebrew. He had also learnt all the odes of Horace by heart, and of course had been through the six books of Euclid and algebra to simple equations!

MEDALSOME

Your mother has 'Jernegan's Lottery Medal.' On it is Minerva holding a spear and a palm branch, standing between a pile of arms and emblems of the arts and sciences. The legend is 'Both hands fill'd for Britain.' In the exergue is 'George reigning,' and a T, for John Sigismund Tanner, who sunk the die. On the reverse is Queen Caroline, crowned, holding a sceptre and watering a grove of young palm trees. The legend is 'Growing arts adorn empire.' In the exergue is Caroline protecting, 1736, and also T for the aforesaid Tanner. Now for the history. Henry Jernegan was the fourth son of Sir Francis Jerningham (the name is the same), of Cossey in Norfolk, and was goldsmith and banker, in Russell Street, Covent Garden. He made a curious silver cistern, which was disposed of by lottery in the year 1737, and of which there is an engraving by Vertue. The price of a ticket was either 5s. or 6s., and the purchaser of each share received into the bargain one of these silver medals, worth about 3s. The medal induced people to buy shares, and about 30,000 of them were struck. Queen Caroline took a few shares.

THE HABITS OF FOREIGNERS

CHINESE CORPSE MOUNTAIN

The White Cloud Mountain is at Canton. It is the Chinese holy of holies, whither the dead bodies are sent from all parts of the world. Frequently fifteen hundred corpses will arrive there in one day. The steamboat company charges forty dollars for the passage of a live Chinaman, and one hundred and sixty dollars for a dead one.

COINS OF THE REALMS

There are one thousand Portuguese reis in four shillings, and two thousand Brazilian reis in three shillings and elevenpence. There are a hundred centavos in ninepence-halfpenny. There are a hundred Austrian kreuzers in one shilling and tenpence. There are sixteen Indian annas in one shilling and eightpence. There are five hundred Belgian, French, Italian, or Swiss centimes in four shillings. There are a hundred Russian kopecks in two shillings and threepence. There are three hundred German pfennigs in two shillings and elevenpence. You will find a good list in the Postal Guide. The values vary with the rate of exchange, but of course very slightly in such small amounts.

MILES AND MILES

What is a mile? Well, an English mile has 1,760 yards, and an English geographical mile has 2,025 yards. An Arabian mile, however, has 2,148 yards; while a mile in Bohemia contains 10,137. A mile in Brabant has 6,082, in Burgundy 6,183; in China the lis has 629. The Danish mile has 8,244 yards, while the Dutch has 8,101, and the Flemish 6,869. The French league has 4,860 yards, the French marine league has 6,075, while there is a land league (not an Irish one) with 4,263. A German mile has 10,126 yards when it is 'long,' and 6,859 when it is 'short,' and 8,100 when it is 'geographical.' A mile in Hamburg contains 8,244 yards, in Hanover 11,559, in Hungary 9,110. In Ireland there are 2,240 yards, in Italy 2,025. The Persian parasang has 6,086 yards. The Poles have a short mile of 6,071 yards, and a long one with 8,130. The Portuguese lequas contains 6,768 yards. The Prussian mile has 8,462 yards; the old Roman mile has either 1,615 or 1,628 yards; the modern Roman mile has 2,027; the Russian verst has 1,169 yards; the Saxon mile 9,904; the Scotch 1,984; and the Silesian 7,086. The Spaniards have two leagues, one of 7,415 yards, another of 4,636 only. A Swedish mile has 11,703 yards, and a Turkish one 1,826. Here we must stop; and now – what is a mile on the Continent? Next time you hear that a friend has been driving his tricycle at ten miles an hour through Germany, you may be quite sure they were not Hanoverian ones.

ALARM ROPE

Yes, it may be occasionally done, even now, but years ago, before railways were extended, the practice must have been much more general with the Eastern couriers. Here is the modus operandi as we have seen it described: When one of these men, so tired with a long tramp that he is glad to lie down on the open ground, and perhaps under a burning sun, determines to take a short nap, it is very necessary that he should adopt some means to prevent his oversleeping himself. So he unwinds a portion of a rope which he carries wrapped round his ankle, and slipping it between the toes of one of his naked feet, he draws out the end beyond his foot to what he considers a proper length for his purpose. The rope is made of some substance which will burn very regularly and slowly, and so the courier pulls out as much as he thinks will burn for an hour, or half an hour, or as long as he wishes to sleep, and sets fire to the end of it. Then he lies down and takes his nap, feeling sure that when the rope burns close to his toe he will wake up quickly enough.

Chapter 3

'A DOCTOR MIGHT HELP YOU. WE CANNOT'

Health and disease among 'Our Boys'

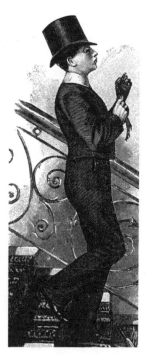

THE average B.O.P. reader – to judge by most of the illustrations, anyway – was reasonably affluent, and usually a public-schoolboy, wearing a natty selection of top-hats and stiff collars.

But the B.O.P. often tried to show that it was aimed at all boys of *every* social group. Dr Gordon Stables, R.N. who wrote regularly on health and fitness, took pains to emphasise his own working class credentials:

> This article [*he wrote, in* A New Year's Letter to Working Lads] is intended for my real working-bees of boys, whose life, I know for a fact, is hard to bear at times. And although I may be accused sometimes of writing only for school 'chaps' and young Eton 'toffs,' I really have all classes high and low in my mind when I give advice. And I have a soft side even to mill-hands and miners.

It is claimed that Stables invented the caravan, at least the first purpose-built leisure caravan, made specially for him in Bristol and in which he travelled the length of the land, which facilitated his desire to meet lower as well as higher-class boys:

> While passing through Lancashire, etc, in my 'Wanderer,' through squalid villages and along dusty roads, which stopped not until I reached Staleybridge, I received no end of favours and courtesy from many a smutty-faced but kind-hearted fellow who knew me but as a gentleman gipsy.

Although married and a father, Stables was an admirer of the healthy, muscular, young male body, judging by the reminiscences of his own boyhood that he shared with his readers:

> There never was a boy yet, I do believe, who did not envy and admire brawn and muscle, perhaps even more than brain. At school I know, when I was a youth, the lads who could strip well by the mill-damside, when we were going in for a swim were

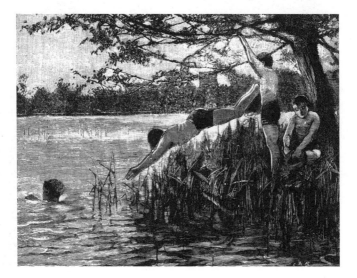

kings of the castle. As far, too, as my experience extends, pluck always goes hand in hand with a well-developed chest and a Highland leg. [*The 'Highland leg', whatever that may be, crops up regularly in some of the* Answers to Correspondents.] Let me see now. There comes up before my mind's eye, as I write, a vision of days gone by. It is a little lake of water, with birch-clad braes rising up at one side of it, and a hill at the other, covered with golden gorse and musical with the songs of linnet and thrush – the lintie and the mavis. It is a lovely afternoon in early summer, and on the brink of the little, dark, deep loch stand, or squat, six of us schoolboys. We have been bathing and swimming and splashing and laughing till the very 'welkin' rang again with the glad and gleeful sound of our voices. We have finished 'a Roman race' as we called it, round the lake, and are dressing. We haven't got much on yet, because we have been taking stock of each other's form – measuring legs, feeling arms, trying hard knuckles, and so forth.

Such passages today read a little creepily, but whatever Stables' motives, the consistent theme of all his advice to boys was of purity, cleanliness, muscularity, bravery and stamina, usually achieved through copious use of a cold bath in the morning.

In one article Stables took some effort to show that this was a procedure that boys of any class could find time for, even those who had had to start work at the age of twelve or thirteen instead of lounging around in public school classrooms:

Says a courteous correspondent, 'How can a lad have a morning tub who starts work at 6 a.m.? Thousands where I work never know what a bath before breakfast is. This bath they never see. The breakfast they take in a beer can, and there is no time for recreation.'

Well, I thought of these words this morning when I awoke at 5 a.m., my usual hour.

'Now,' I said, 'I shall time myself, with no unusual hurry.'

I got up, lit my lamp and looked at the clock. Remember, the 'tub' with the big sponge in it was ready and waiting. I stripped off all the garments of night, and kneeling down before the sitz bath, soaped and well washed face, arms, and chest. Then in I got, sponged all over, dried with one towel and rough-rubbed with another. Dressed myself in knickerbockers suit, just as a country gentleman should, combed and brushed my hair, brushed my teeth and stood ready for a long day's work. Now for the time – eleven minutes and a half! Had I had only to throw on a workman's suit I could have done it in ten minutes. I felt fresh as a daisy, had a draught of water, and then, lantern in hand, set off away down through the grounds to the wigwam where I work, and had to go back for breakfast at eight, after seeing to my great dogs.

Looking back a hundred years or more, I find it difficult to see any medical rationale for many of Stables' recommendations. Certainly, his ideas of how the body works were more akin to those of a fringe therapist than someone who had done a medical training:

I wish to draw your attention to the fact that not only is the heart muscular, but so is one of the coats of the stomach, and intestinal canal also... the muscular coat of the stomach being weak, digestion is feebly performed, the blood becomes thin and watery because it is imperfectly fed, every organ of the body loses tone in consequence, the bowels become irregular in their action, the breathing or staying powers are lowered, the heart flutters as it beats out the blood that it seems heartily ashamed of, the nerves are starved, and all kinds of trouble, real and imaginary, is generated.

The symptoms of such a bodily or blood condition are not the same in all. Your fat boy degenerates into a nag of unwholesome tallow, spiritless and unambitious; your lanky lad becomes a little old woman in boy's clothes, with all an old woman's whims, and even more. Both perhaps are troubled with bad dreams at night, while from a state of over-selfconsciousness by day, their lives are miserable enough in all conscience.

Now about 90 per cent of boys suffer more or less from the symptoms I have roughly outlined, and the worst of it is that their parents, instead of taking a commonsense view of the matter, usually jump to the conclusion it is medicine the lads want, and either apply to the apothecary or dose them as they think right, with tonics, fish-oil, and all sorts of garbage, which would best be poured down a rat's hole.

Stables was the mainstay of the health and fitness advice dished out in articles and in the *Answers*, and he promised unique benefits if boys followed his advice. 'I will tell you,' he wrote, 'how to get rid of the trifling but troublesome complaints of boyhood so that when you grow men you will be strong enough to roll over a bullock on the emu plains of Australia with one blow from your fist – more or less.'

(As we'll see in another chapter, the ability to kill animals cleanly as well as look after them was one that the British boy was encouraged to cultivate.)

In the answers that follow, in spite of the occasional shakiness of the advice, there seem to be two guiding – and good – principles. First, the policy of the B.O.P., perhaps ahead of its time, was to advise against all 'quacks' and quack medicines, at a time when the less reputable publications often made their money by carrying advertisements for such remedies:

Do not, if you value your future welfare, be led to put your trust in quack medicines.

– oOo –

You'll get better as you grow older if you read and go by Dr. Gordon Stables' advice in our paper, 'Health and Athletics.' Read back. The pamphlets are *quackery.*

– oOo –

The Scarborough man is an arrant quack. Do not read such books. Consult a practising physician.

– oOo –

Do not read those thrice-accursed quack pamphlets. They emanate from the vilest scoundrels that hanging would be too good for. Lead a life of thought-purity. Sleep on a hard mattress with little bed-clothing. Take quinine and iron for a month; exercise, cold bath, and good society. This will soon free you from all nervousness and make a man of you.

The second sensible stance taken by the B.O.P. was that if there was ever a danger that the correspondent had a serious problem, the reply – sometimes with some urgency – advised the writer to see a doctor as soon as possible. In fact, in terms of the usefulness of the advice, that was probably all it usually offered – the range of answers is more interesting for what it reveals about boys' preoccu-pations than as a source of self-help:

SO WHITE IN THE FACE – Iron. Best form, bi-palatinoids. Are you a girl? Don't like your writing. You wouldn't do for our private clerk. It is too undecided.

– oOo –

We counsel wearing belts, not braces, which give a boy shoulders like a soda-water bottle.

– oOo –

The snail remedy for eczema is one of the commonest we have, and has been practised by the country folks for centuries. The only wonderful thing about the cure is the ignorance which calls it new. It is as well known as a cobweb for a cut finger. Any cool slimy substance would probably have the same effect.

– oOo –

The continued drinking of hot water is certainly most injurious.

– o O o –

No, if you feel strong enough take all and every form of exercise except thinking too much. That is about the only exercise that hurts nervous boys like you.

– o O o –

Only a surgeon can treat bow legs. You cannot do so yourself.

– o O o –

With some people, gaping is sympathetic; it may arise from habit or from fatigue. In the first case, conquer your habit; in the second, go to bed! But it is not a very dreadful malady after all.

– o O o –

Follow the advice of your doctor. You will never be eligible for Government employment, and had better give up all thoughts of volunteering. Never talk to strangers of your ailments, or be guided by the advice they give.

– o O o –

A doctor might help you. We cannot.

– o O o –

A Scotch schoolboy is a lad of a different type, and here again we cannot speak positively. It sounds pretty stiff to begin work at 6 a.m., breakfast at 8, walk 2^1/$_2$ miles to school at 9, get home at 3, and work straight away to midnight. Cases are on record where such intense application has been continued for years; but we should think for a growing lad that a little less study, a little more exercise, and a little more sleep, would not in any way decrease the amount of knowledge he would acquire, and would be more conducive to his health. It certainly would be better for the majority of boys.

– o O o –

COLD BATH – Before breakfast in the morning is the best time. Get up earlier.

– o O o –

PIGEON-BREAST – Caused by a tendency to rickets. If it is a positive deformity it would prevent you from entering the service. You cannot alter it after the bones are set.

– o O o –

DIZZINESS – Consult a doctor. It is a nasty symptom.

– o O o –

Consult a surgeon, and do so *soon.*

– o O o –

Fiddlesticks! Your legs cannot be too big. Perhaps you are Scotch!

– o O o –

HARRIER – Has hairs on arms and legs, moles, blotches, and maggots on face, fat legs, big feet and knees, and is short-winded. Poor HARRIER! Exercise. Follow the harriers.

– o O o –

JUMBO – Heigho! Indian clubs, O Jumbo! are elongated dumb-bells. They are not insurance societies! You will find nothing in our articles about an Indian's 'expectation of life,' but you may discover a health-giving exercise for your policy-

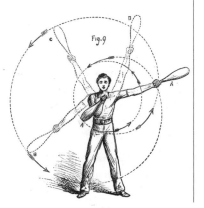

holders, and so we give the information you ask for. The articles on Indian Clubs were in the August and September parts for 1882.

– o O o –

If your legs are getting bent at nineteen years of age, you had perhaps better see a doctor. Probably he will change your diet, and give you some such tonic as Parrish's Chemical Food.

– o O o –

SPASMODIC WINKING – It is a most disagreeable nervous complaint. You must attend well to general health, and now and then take a course of cod-liver oil, with citrate of iron and quinine. You will derive much benefit from the cold morning tub. Write again and tell us how you are. We like to shake hands with friends across the Herring Pond.

– o O o –

Jamie wants a cure for his leg bending at the knee. We hope Jamie, and all our other boys, bend the knee every night. Parrish's Chemical Food, a teaspoonful thrice a day in water, or Fellow's Syrup will strengthen bones.

– o O o –

JOB and his friends must, we fear, put up with their boils, or else apply to a doctor.

– o O o –

SUPERFLUOUS HAIR – Leave it alone. If you do not, you may repent it in after life.

– o O o –

WEAK WRISTS – No, gymnastics will not make big bones. Try Fellows syrup, a teaspoonful thrice daily in water at meal-times. At nineteen the bones are within a few years of being fully formed.

– o O o –

No; avoid it by all means. Chewing cocae leaves becomes a habit from which there is no getting over.

– o O o –

No; the common-sense practice of ventriloquism cannot injure the health.

– o O o –

Removing moles is dangerous.

– o O o –

See a surgeon; all interference by yourself is dangerous.

– o O o –

Sleeping with a pad between knees and feet strapped tends to straighten legs bent in, but you had better see a doctor.

– o O o –

Soap or grease your feet, and you will avoid blisters. In the last war the Germans wore no socks, but used a square piece of soft linen saturated with tallow and wrapped around the foot. [*Probably the Franco-Prussian War of 1870.*]

– o O o –

HEADACHE – Something radically wrong. Consult a doctor at once.

– o O o –

Surely the proof of the training should be in the running! If you can live on bacon and ham, and win your race, what more do you want? If, however, you study any method except your own, you will find such things, like all other salt and fatty meats, strongly condemned.

– o O o –

Take the lead out of your mouth; it can do you no good, and may perhaps poison you. To keep the mouth moist some people suck a small flint pebble, but even this practice is not recommended, and is absolutely dangerous when running, or indulging in violent exercise.

– o O o –

TALL BOY – The delay will, we fear, render the answer useless, although it is given at the earliest moment. The London address of the manageress of the Ventnor Convalescent Home is at 12, Pall Mall, S.W. We never answer medical queries.

– o O o –

The drowsiness of an evening of which you complain, in regard to your studies for examination, is, supposing you are in fair health, not by any means a matter to be attacked, as you would seem to think, with medicine. It may be simply a sign that you are honestly wearied, and thus Nature's call to rest. You might try a short, sharp walk; but, whatever you do, eschew stimulants or drugs. Nature, if thus forced, is sure to take reprisals; and to force the jaded mind inevitably implies reaction.

– o O o –

The optician you name used to live in the Strand, but he is dead.

– o O o –

The subject is really a medical one, and for it you should consult a doctor. There are many books on corpulency; one, a cheap pamphlet by Banting, obtainable of Messrs. Harrison, Pall Mall, would give you a great many useful hints. Meat is not necessarily fattening, but tea, if taken too frequently, will be apt to ruin your digestion.

– o O o –

The very distressing complaint which you mention is mostly caused by indigestion. There is no reason why it should not be stopped, or rather removed. As to the best mode of removing it, consult a duly qualified medical man.

– o O o –

G. S. – This boy bites his finger-nails, and wants a cure. Punch would say, 'Don't.' This advice is good, but not complete enough. G.S. might have his hands tied behind his back. That would do it. Or let him wear gloves and smear the finger-tips with mustard; or, better still, wear a respirator studded with needles, the points to the front. Next!

– o O o –

MATCH STALK – Twenty years

hence you will be thankful you were as you now describe yourself. Sturdy boyhood often means corpulent manhood. Rise early, exercise freely, work hard, walk much, and feed wholesomely and regularly.

– oOo –

CAUSE OF WARTS – Warts are of various sorts (we may give a little sermon on them one day); but the ordinary hard wart is really a species of corn. Decomposing animal matter is said to favour their growth. Probably the blood is below par when many warts grow. Take ten drops of tincture of iron in water thrice daily.

– oOo –

A WRINKLE (Marcus) – We cannot tell you, Marcus, how to remove your solitary wrinkle; but as you are one of our boys, we hope you'll live to have lots more!

– oOo –

AFFLICTED ONE – We have never heard of a cure.

– oOo –

NO CALF ON HIS LEG – Well, do not wear knicks till the calf comes. Exercise will do it. Behold a Highlander's leg. How does he get it, think you? Why, by climbing hills.

– oOo –

THE FLAT MAC – You *are* a flat, Master Mac. Acetic acid put on the head would remove hair, and scalp and all, as clean and clear as knife of Indian. Who said your brain was softening? It seems to us you were born so.

– oOo –

KILLING WILD BEASTS – You are a funny lad. Where are you going, anyhow? What sort of wild beasts are you going to kill – weasels or walruses? It is a pity Barnum has gone, he might have let you have a shy at one of his lions ... Your hot, red nose probably proceeds from dyspepsia, but it might really be advantageous in killing wild beasts – frighten them, you know!

– oOo –

You have our sympathy, but we are unable to offer advice in such matters. Where the most skilled doctors, with an intimate knowledge of the case, have failed, it is not for an outsider to succeed.

– oOo –

CHALKY ... who 'measures a little too much round his stomach,' is recommended not to eat so much. If for 'stomach' we are to read 'chest,' we congratulate him, and trust that, so far from 'lessening' it, he will increase it. No boy can be too broad-chested.

– oOo –

TOOTHACHE – It is a sad affliction. it is a pity, however, to take out a tooth that can be filled. Bunter's Nervine often gives magical relief. Beware of so-called Yankee dentists. They are not all bad – but ...

– oOo –

THE MOST UNLUCKY LAD LIVING – Seventeen years old, pale faced and pimply, cut his moustache with the scissors and wants a pal. His only comfort is the B.O.P. Well don't die yet awhile, old man. Take iron, as recommended to Arrandoon. Also the cold tub. The pal will come in time. Meanwhile suppose you make pals with dumbbells for half an hour every morning before breakfast!

– oOo –

Steadfastly and persistently resolve that you will not blink, and you will find that the power of the will will eventually prove strong enough to master the muscles. It is absurd to suppose that you now bear the character of being thick-headed and lazy solely because you cannot leave off blushing. Try and discover the other reasons.

– oOo –

HEALTH – We do not know how to pulverise earthworms, but can quite understand that a mouthful of such muck would effectually clear out everything – hollow tooth and all. Many are the cures we have heard for toothache, but yours is the nastiest.

– oOo –

MAKING THE CALVES GROW – You silly boy! Was the poultice you put on your back made of Scotch oatmeal? You make us laugh. Try exercise, climb hills, ride the cycle, swim, and eat the oatmeal.

– oOo –

Clean your teeth twice a day instead of twice a week.

– oOo –

'Will dyeing my hair from white to black cause insanity?' Well, we should not advise you to try, judging from the character of this and your other questions, we think that there would be some risk in your case, and we would earnestly recommend you to refrain for the future even from the mild excitement of writing foolish questions to an editor.

– o O o –

Numbness, especially if accompanied by whiteness of the fingers, shows that you have been in the water too long.

– o O o –

The blanching of the extremities is probably a sign that you have been quite long enough in the water. Some constitutions do not admit of immersion for any length of time. We cannot tell you of anything to prevent it, and you would do well promptly to take heed of nature's warning.

– o O o –

You will never find it too often to bathe once a day.

– o O o –

You are the first blushing politician we have come across. The BOY'S OWN PAPER does not attempt to be a newspaper; we left that side of the subject for others to take up, and we shall do as much as we can to keep clear of party questions and political matters. If you become much of a politician you will soon leave off blushing.

– o O o –

Get more roomy boots, that is all you can do.

– o O o –

Tightly fitting machine-made boots mean, as we daily see and hear, a corned and bunioned nation.

– o O o –

There is only one certain cure for drunkenness, and that is total abstention from alcoholic liquors. No black draughts or chemists' compounds will ever frighten a man from intoxication. If he is too weak-willed to moderate his desire for strong drink, the only thing he can do to save himself is to abandon it altogether.

– o O o –

CHEEKY – See how your query looks in print! 'Would you be kind enough to tell me what I could do to get rid of my fat cheeks?" Eat less, and think more.

– o O o –

FATTIE, F.H., and Others – We do not know the degree of 'skinniness' to which you severally wish to attain. Eating vinegar with a fork is reputed to produce spareness and sharpness. Perhaps a few days of such diet might have a desirable effect on both your bodily and mental powers, and open your eyes to the absurdity of troubling us with such questions.

– o O o –

LEWIS – Well really! There is no satisfying some people! We will pass you on as you are. 'Dear Editor: – I am extremely fat, and I want to no how I can get it down. Please put it in the Correspondence. I hopes you won't put Think less and eat more, or any other absurdness, which is your usual. I am, etc.' Where did we tell you to eat more and think less O Lewis? Is that what you have been trying to do?

– o O o –

SIMPLE SYMAN – 'I have joined a Mutual Improvement class. Last Tuesday evening a reading was

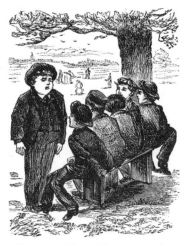

'I say, you fellows! Can't you make room for a little one?'

given by one of the members, and we all had to criticise it in turn; but when my turn came round I coloured up, and sat trembling in my seat. 'Now then, Syman,' said the chairman. I rose and stammered out something, and then sat down amidst the uproarious laughter of the class. Is there anything I can do to prevent this unpleasant feeling?' It seems to us that these fellows have acted very wisely in going in for improvement, for they are obviously much in need of it. Try again, Syman, and you will soon get over your nervousness!

– o O o –

Consult a doctor at once. It would be a pity your figure should be spoiled. Your proportions are splendid for your age.

– oOo –

Stammerers are quite unsuited for a seafaring life. You have no more chance of serving on a merchant-man than on a Queen's ship. Even a penny steamboat would come to grief under a captain who had to take refuge in 'Gug-gug-gug-g-g-go a-a-a-a-st-tut-tut-tut-tarn!'

– oOo –

VOX FAUCIBUS HAESIT – informs us that he cured himself of stammering by shutting himself up in a dark room where he was sure no one could hear him, and then talking out loud just fast enough to permit of his correctly pronounc-ing every word he uttered.

– oOo –

We agree with your manager that your stammering is only habit. We also think that if you were to make up your mind to get rid of it, and refrained from treating it as inevitable, that you would soon learn to talk like other people.

– oOo –

YELLOW TEETH – Too late, we fear. You have been using patent tooth powders till you have destroyed the enamel. You cannot restore the gilt to the gingerbread, or the lacquer to the brass. Use only soap and soft water, or a little carbonate of soda.

– oOo –

Do not trouble about your voice; you are simply passing through the usual experience of youth. Do not attempt to sing or otherwise force it at present, and a year hence you will probably have nothing to complain of.

– oOo –

VOICE NOT CHANGED YET – Well, you must exercise the vocal cords by reading aloud daily in your own room. Read and recite. It is your only chance. Are you tall and thin?

– oOo –

The coals you have managed to get into your hands ought to be picked out with a fine needle.

– oOo –

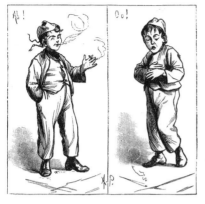

The Beginning   *and*   The End
(and serve him well right, too!)

Occasionally the Editor, and/or Dr Stables, 'got it right'. The B.O.P. was an early antagonist of smoking among boys, not because of any foreknowledge of the carcinogenic or cardiovascular effects, but more, perhaps, because it was an adult pleasure and boys were not adults.

To reinforce the message, the B.O.P. presented the results of survey of the habits of leading sportsmen, reporting that 'the majority of Queen's Prize winners at Wimbledon, most of the leading oarsmen, including Trickett and Hanlan, and those crack Yankee shots, Mr. Partello and Dr. Carver, consider the less stimulants and narcotics a human being indulges in, the better for his physical health.' The message was spoilt somewhat by the news that 'Private Rae, Queen's Prize winner in 1878, confesses that he indulges to the extent of two ounces of tobacco per week, and "a glass sometimes," but he has nevertheless the courage to maintain that both forms of indulgence are reprehensible, and that he would be much better if he gave them up entirely.' The survey, says the B.O.P., presents 'a consensus of authoritative opinion that leaves no room for doubt.' And the message was gravely hammered home, week after week, in *Answers to Correspondents*:

Smoking may perhaps do some men no harm, but it rarely does them any good, and it is especially prejudicial in the case of growing lads, for various well-understood physiological reasons.

– oOo –

There can be no question as to the injurious effects of tobacco on growing lads; and in training tobacco is always strictly forbidden. 2. The principal narcotics in use in various quarters of the globe are – alcohol, opium, tobacco, chloral, absinthe, haschisch, coca leaf, betel nut, intoxicating fungus, kava. 3. The address of the 'English Anti-Tobacco Society' – from whom you will doubtless be able to obtain all the information you desire on the subject – is 26, Corporation Street, Manchester. Mr. Reade is the secretary. 4. Dr. Richardson, F.R.S., who has gone into the matter fully, thus sums up: 'Smoking tobacco in every form, is a habit better not acquired, and when acquired is better abandoned. The young should specially avoid the habit. It gives a doubtful pleasure for a certain penalty.' Our own opinion runs very decidedly in the same direction.

– oOo –

PIPES – There is such a disease. It generally comes from smoking wooden pipes. The mouth gets inflamed, then a sore rises, and this gradually leads to quite a cancer forming in the lip or cheek.

– oOo –

An excellent notion! We hope you will keep your promise never to touch tobacco unless you make it yourself out of the one plant you are so proud of. Grow your own tobacco, cure your own tobacco, and smoke your own tobacco; and then send us on the report from your medical attendant!

– oOo –

No wonder you are lanky. A boy of fourteen *smoking*. What will you be at thirty, *if* you live?

– oOo –

Yes; of course it prevents development of body by weakening the heart and brain. Writing beautiful.

– oOo –

The receipt is useless and mischievous. Smoking will weaken your heart and interfere with your growth in strength. If you want to grow up lanky, pale, and with blood as thin as an old wife's third cup of tea, smoke by all means. If you want a pimply face, smoke. If you want to have no more brains than a bladder of lard, smoke.

– oOo –

Yes, it will hinder you in body and mind. No one has any right to

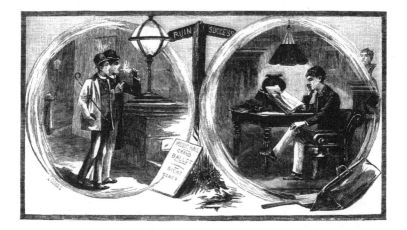

smoke unless he is subject to grief, care, and worry, or hard work. Besides, tobacco breeds care of its own, and causes weakness of heart and head in the young.

– oOo –

Smoke rises in the air, therefore smoke is lighter than the air, there-fore if you fill yourself with smoke you decrease your weight. Therefore, though the effect of two cigarettes a week is not, strictly speaking, enormous, still it must have a tendency to elevatory influence and would not diminish the lightheartedness that troubles you; therefore we say don't do it.

Perhaps the most frequent topic of concern for Dr Stables was one which was never referred to directly but hinted at by various euphemisms. In one of his many articles for the BOY'S OWN PAPER, Stables wrote 'a word of solemn warning to all young men who may have acquired habits that are prejudicial to health. The strug-gle to get free will be a terrible one; but if they do not succeed there is only unhappiness in store for them.'

In this delicate area, without being able to read the boys' actual questions, it's difficult sometimes to know exactly what everyone was on about. Eating fatty foods? Injecting heroin? Playing chicken on the railway line? They are all habits prejudicial to health but clearly, in this case, it is the looming temptations of adolescence that Stables and his stable of advisers are on about. The Rev. E. J. Hardy, M. A. 'Chaplain to H. M. Forces', gets a little more explicit in his article *We Shall All Grow Up,* when he writes about 'the tyrant of impurity':

> How he must tremble when he sees a boy refusing to listen to nasty stories, not polluting his mind with unclean thoughts, and turning away his eyes from books and pictures at which he would not like his mother to see him looking!

(The Rev. Hardy wrote a book called *How to be Happy though Married,* so we are entitled to think that he was a bit of a misanthrope, or at least a misogynist.)

In the light of the references to reading matter and its arousing effects, it's quite a shock to come across a picture of bare breasts in one issue. (And I don't mean the goat udders being tweaked in Volume 9).

At the bottom of page 621 of Volume 3 is a young lady, barely out of her teens – visibly so – looking the reader straight in the eyes with her naked breasts in full view.

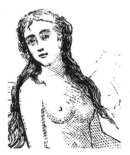

It's only the rest of her body from the waist down that gives licence to this otherwise shocking breach of all that the B.O.P. stands for. She is in fact a mermaid, and unlike Hans Christian Anderson's *Little Mermaid* in the Disney film of that name which was to be produced a hundred years later, she is not wearing a bikini.

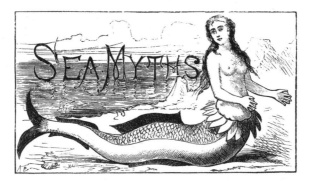

Regardless of her icthyological undergarments, it's difficult to imagine that this wasn't seen by the Religious Tract Society as a breach of propriety, and certainly I have come across no other semi-nude female in other issues, search as I might.

There were many moral tales warning against impurity scattered through the columns of the BOY'S OWN PAPER, in addition to the high tone of the serials and stories. This one was called *Words that Stain:*

> A small brush of camel's hair had been dipped into a fluid in which was some nitrate of silver, or 'caustic,' as it is sometimes called. The brush was wiped upon a white sheet. Pretty soon there appeared a black stain upon a white surface. It did not look very dark at first, but the action of the light seemed to deepen the colour, until it was an ugly spot that could not be washed out nor bleached out in a whole summer's sunshine. A bright lad heard a vile word and an impure story. He thought them over. They became fixed in his memory, and they left a stain which could not be washed out by all the waters of this great round earth. Don't lend your ears to be defiled. In these days of bad books it is our duty to take care what we read. A bad story smirches the heart, pollutes the memory, and inflames the fancy. Shun these things as you would poisonous vipers, and ask God to help you.

What Would Mother Say?, by the Rev. A. N. Malan, forges together Christianity and motherhood in a powerful blow for purity:

> Do you ever dare, when alone, or with one or two companions, to do anything you would be ashamed to do in your mother's presence? Look honestly into the matter. Remember that God is now searching you through – that you cannot dare dissemble with him – that he is reading your inmost soul as clearly as you can read an open book.
>
> The boy who has a pure and true idea of reverence for his mother is never left to himself. Her presence occupies a chamber in his heart. He bears her remembrance about with him – as the high priest bore about with him the remembrance of the people by the engraved gems of his breastplate. In moment of privacy, in the time of temptation, when some evil thought has arisen, some wicked word has been spoken, some sinful action has been suggested – if a boy reverences his mother, her sacred presence rises before him, and in the strength of her remembrance there comes the preventing power of the Holy Spirit; and he has courage to resist the devil, and comes out of the temptation with unsullied conscience.

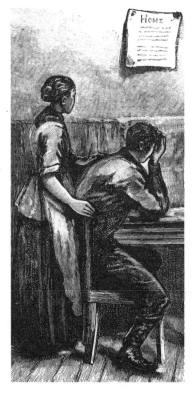

And the 'mother' card is played in some of the *Answers to Correspondents*:

We are thoroughly ashamed of you. You must know that it is wrong. Would you dare to tell your father or mother of it?

– oOo –

In a paper read not only by boys of all ages, but also largely by their sisters, the difficulty of effectively treating on such a subject will be readily understood. While, however, it is impossible for us to go into details, we trust the whole tone and teaching of our paper must warn and tell against impurity of every kind, whether of thought, word, or deed. At school, as elsewhere, it is a safe rule to avoid everything, no matter who may be the tempter, of which you could not fearlessly speak to your father or mother.

Probably it was assumed that even if the boy had not written about masturbation he was doing it anyway and it would do no harm to tell him to stop. Like William Acton, author of the mid-19th century book, *The Functions and Disorders of the Reproductive Organs*, the BOY'S OWN PAPER editorial staff almost certainly believed – or behaved as if they believed – that 'In a state of health no sexual impression should ever affect a child's mind or body. All its vital energy should be employed in building up the growing frame, in storing up external impressions, and educating the brain to receive them. During a well-regulated childhood, and in the case of ordinary temperaments, there is no temptation to infringe this primary law of nature.'

Well, clearly, among the readers of the B.O.P. there were many who had had neither a well-regulated childhood, nor an ordinary temperament:

Give up bad habits, and get a Harness's Electropathic Belt.

– oOo –

MISERABLE – We are glad that by following our advice you are Miserable now no longer. We wish other boys would abjure all evil habits, and go in for more exercise, the bath, good food, wholesome reading, and hard bed or mattress, and if medicine be needed, just about 10 to 15 drops of tincture of iron thrice daily in water after meals.

– o O o –

ANOTHER CONVERT FOR GORDON STABLES – Well, we are glad you are. Stick to the bath and exercise. Never think evil, far less act it, and you will sleep better and grow up a big strong happy man.

– o O o –

EGROEG – Bravo! lad. We like you, though you do spell your name upside down. You've been taking our advice and you're the better for it. How we wish all our boys would do the same. You'll be a man yet.

– o O o –

Glad you are penitent. We trust in time. Obey all the laws of health. Be out of doors all you can. Read good books. Keep good company. For medicine, a teaspoonful of Fellow's Syrup twice a day in water after meals. Avoid quacks and keep your thoughts pure. Take a cold bath every morning with a handful of sea-salt in it dissolved overnight.

– o O o –

Your ailments are almost wholly imaginary, and you must have written to quacks, who have been seeking to trade on your fears. Never again relapse into the hateful habit; take as much outdoor exercise as you can conveniently command, and if you do not already do so, take a cold douche bath (or failing that sponge yourself with cold water) every morning. The symptoms that you deem so alarming are common to almost all whose health wants tone, and need not worry you. For a week or so you might, perhaps take some simple tonic, but above all keep good hours, be temperate in all things, and let the advertising sharks alone.

– o O o –

BAD DREAMS – To some extent they are natural but not to any great extent. Better consult a doctor.

– o O o –

MORE BAD DREAMS – Any cause for your bad dreams? If so, remove it, as you value your future welfare.

– o O o –

Throw the pamphlet straightway into the fire, and avoid the writer of it as you would your worst enemy. Simply give up at once and for ever the baleful practice, and seeking help in this, as in all other matters, from God, feel thankful that you wrote to us before committing yourself to the tender mercies of the cruel advertising sharks.

– o O o –

Pray give up all such monstrous notions. Surely Christ is able, not only to forgive us our sins, but also to keep us from falling! How dare one think of mutilating the body God has given rather than ask Him for restraining and upholding grace? Live plainly, eschewing alcohol and smoking, retire and rise early, take a cold bath every morning, and engage as actively as possible in some good outdoor sport.

– o O o –

The only recipe needful is – give up the hateful practice at once and for ever; and if the general health has suffered, consult any respectable medical practitioner, and avoid as you would your worst enemies the cruel advertising sharks.

– o O o –

Beware of bad habits, or your life is not worth sixpence.

– o O o –

Give up the sinful habit at once and for ever; take as much outdoor exercise as possible, with cold bath every morning, and some good tonic. Read our recent articles on Health and Athletics.

– o O o –

If you are to read Shakespeare solely for the harm you can get from it, pray leave it alone. There is no book in this world you cannot turn to evil purposes if you are so minded.

– o O o –

No good. Do not take medicine at all. Just live well and exercise plenty. Whenever you begin to think disagreeable thoughts get a book and read. [*But not Shakespeare, presumably.*]

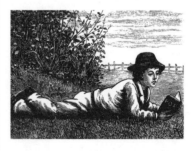

– o O o –

If you now entirely abstain from the evil practices you mention, and take good food and regular exercise – which, being in the army, you will have to, of course – you may escape from sure evil.

– o O o –

Do not despair. Trust in God and you may yet be well. You are unfortunately an example of a numerous class of lads who ruin their health by evil practices and find it out when almost too late. Consult and trust in your own doctor.

– o O o –

Read reply to 'Despair.' Take an iron tonic, cold bath, and Kepler's Extract of Malt, a dessertspoonful thrice a day. If you love your life, beware. You know what is meant.

– o O o –

It is sad that one so young as you should ask such a question. But you are but one of many 'troubled ones,' therefore we answer you. Yes, life will be worth living if you can at once and for ever give up the evil habit. We call it by a mild term. Follow the rules of health as laid down plainly by Dr. Gordon Stables in his paper, 'Athletics and Health.' Live a pure life in thought and deed, and *pray* for Divine help.

– o O o –

Well, it is your own fault though we feel sorry. Do not despair. As regards your bad habits, it is a matter of almost life or death.

– o O o –

If to any great extent, what you speak of is dangerous, and you must consult a doctor. The other boy is a blackguard, and his habits will lead him to a life of great misery. To some extent what you mention is natural. Keep pure and pray for strength.

– o O o –

The worst thing a boy can do, bar one. It will weaken your heart and head, and whiten your face as well.

– o O o –

Of course you are. Smoking is bad enough, but the other is a thousand times worse. You are killing yourself.

– o O o –

You may do much good by taking a cold bath every morning with a handful or two of sea-salt in it. also Fellow's Syrup of the Phosphates, a teaspoonful in water thrice daily. Give up bad habits, looking to the <u>Strong</u> for strength, or your life is not worth many years' purchase.

– o O o –

Come, now, let us have some of that confidence. Isn't it yourself and not your brother who have done wrong and are suffering. Try the cold bath, cod-liver oil, outdoor exercise, and purity of mind and body.

– oOo –

You must consult your own doctor, and soon. Dr Gordon Stables is pleased that you and hundreds of others appreciate his little sermons in 'Doings'. We do not think he means to be hard on city boys. He just speaks the truth and that isn't always palatable.

– oOo –

Give up, or you will kill yourself or turn an imbecile. Take tonics, the bath, cheerful society, and fresh air.

– oOo –

Your case only just proves how hard and unkind it is for parents and teachers not to warn boys of such dangers as you refer to. Yes; you have possibly injured yourself. Consult your father; doctor at once. Be bold. Doctors are kind.

– oOo –

You are not bad at heart, nor in nature, though you have fallen into bad habits. Guard your tongue and *actions.* Never forget that a Power above is able to strengthen our wills when we are at our very weakest. Pray, then; be always praying in thoughts, and even while at work. Remember, too, as you get morally stronger, that he who thinkest he standeth should take heed lest he fall.

And finally, could this bad habit thing cross the species barrier?

Nothing will cure your St. Bernard of the filthy habit he has acquired except reasoning with him, whip in hand. *But* let him have plenty of green vegetables in his food, else you may reason in vain, or he may reason with you – with his teeth.

However harsh many of the replies were, there was an occasional note of sympathy for the unease of adolescent boyhood. Here's the advice of Dr. Stables, admirer of muscles, cold baths and ten mile walks, to boys who might not have fitted his ideal of boyhood:

Perhaps some boy who reads these columns is not so strong in health as he would like to be; he is more puny in chest and limb than other lads of his age. That is no reason, however, why he should not grow up a healthy and powerful young man. And the only medicine I prescribe is this – exercise, and plenty of it, in the open air. But the taking of exercise for the mere sake of taking it, will do you no more good than the convict gets in his daily walk round the prison yard. Exercise, to be good must be pleasurable. And to a certain extent, exciting. And herein consists the beauty of having a hobby, such as that of butterfly hunting, gathering objects of interest, egg-collecting or botanising – you are taking exercise and you are unaware of it; the pure air makes you hungry, the walking or running gives you sound sleep at night, and these combined make you strong. There – I have preached a sermon in a nutshell!

Chapter 4

=====X=====

'...TEA-LEAVES ARE NOT BRITISH...'

Chauvinism and sexism

JUDGING by today's standards, the BOY'S OWN PAPER and its writers were sexist, racist snobs. Some of the attitudes expressed in its stories, articles and *Answers to Correspondents* would produce gasps of distaste if they were expressed in print nowadays.

So here they come ...

To start with, 'girls', those creatures who are among us but not of us. A boy had sisters and female cousins, as well as mothers and aunts, and he was encouraged by the B.O.P. to treat them with reverence and toleration, while acquiring the belief that they were incapable of much that the average boy was expected to do as a matter of course. The best expression of this attitude in the early years of the magazine comes in an article by a Dr. John Scoffern, whose recipe for exploding spiders was designed to wreak boyish havoc in the average home by terrifying servants and maiden aunts. Scoffern wrote an article describing an 'Electric Pen' invented by Thomas Edison. It was apparently used for drawing on a thin metal plate in such a way that ink could be forced through the holes to reproduce many copies of the drawing.

But the most interesting part of the article is the beginning, where Scoffern treats us to his views of the artistic abilities of girls:

> You will have noticed, if observant, the difference of procedure between a weak amateur artist and a true artist in their respective ways of making a picture. Suppose the picture to be a figure group, for example. The real artist takes his charcoal and rapidly dashes in a general effect and outline, paying due heed to proportion. He does not single out one particular individual in his figure group for special attention, but here a dash, there a line, he treats all alike. He does not think that it is absolutely necessary to begin at a pictorial man's head, and work downwards to the feet, finishing as he goes. His sketch is often rough as rough can be, but he, having apprehended the general cast of his subject rightly, has made no mistake. So far as his sketch goes it is correct; finish will come hereafter.
>
> Contrast this work with the work of a weak amateur, and more especially a weak young lady amateur. She has probably received her artistic instruction – *artistic!* Save the mark! – at some finishing school – I beg her pardon, *college* – where drawing and painting instruction 'in all styles' is professedly taught. She is given a smooth card of tinted paper; she scratches out a sun or moon with a penknife – makes a few trees and gate-posts – all slanting like written letters *l*, and when term vacation comes, takes the thing home for family admiration. In all human accomplishments – I don't adopt the word in the young-ladylike sense of things done, problems solved, aspirations achieved – you will find that success depends on beginning with first principles of sketching (to borrow an artistic mode of expression) before elaborating.
>
> 'Well,' you will exclaim, 'what in the name of wonder has all this rigmarole to do with electric pens?'

Verb sap, as they used to say in B.O.P school stories.

The idea that girls had to be treated differently came to the fore early on when the B.O.P.'s competitions were open to both sexes. (Within a year or so of the B.O.P. starting up, there was a *Girl's Own Paper* and the issue no longer arose.) But when the results of the very first competition were announced, the irksome issue of 'girls' arose. Horror of horrors, after the best two entries, the next best was from Rebecca Isabel Wilson of Notting Hill, clearly a girl. The best entry after that was from Albert Henry Shaw of Huddersfield, but there was no fourth prize, and, peculiarly, it was felt that Albert Henry Shaw should not be done out of the third prize by a girl, so, with what seems to me like trickery of a high order, the Editor decided on the following:

> ... we thought, in the circumstances, it would be fairer to the boy who had won the third prize to give an *extra* prize to the girl who tied second, rather than allow her to displace him. [*Of course, Shaw clearly wasn't the* competitor *who won the third prize.*]

In a regular column called *Doings for the Month*, the writer said:

> Boys go away sometimes and leave their pets to the care of servants. This is wrong. It is best for two boys, or a boy and his sister, to go halves in a fancy, and one 'pard' should always be at home.

A firm rebuff to this idea came in a letter two months later from a female 'pard':

> I venture to remonstrate with the dreadful suggestion which you have made in this month's 'Doings,' to the effect that boys should share their various animals with their sisters, instead of leaving them in the care of servants when they are away at school. Mercifully, in our family we are three sisters; but surely, when

we have to be at matins most mornings through the year at 8.30, and have various other occupations to be attended to through the day, part of the care of two cages of mice, one rat, one bullfinch (and often more), one cage of doves, large aviary (in the garden), three bantams, two aquariums of fishes, one dog, one cat, and very often newts, lizards, salamanders, chameleons, tortoises, and even at one time a hedgehog, surely part of the care of these animals during the term when the boys are away may rest upon the servants. And if these animals are to be *shared* with us, it only means we must also give half the money towards them, make half their cages, and share half the responsibility too. And as we have four brothers, and all have different tastes about animals, we shall be utterly overwhelmed if they take up your suggestion, and offer to share their creature with us. I did go in once for bringing up two puppies with a baby's bottle, and they throve pretty well; but when I got to love them, and they to love me, they were given away, because they were not mine altogether.'

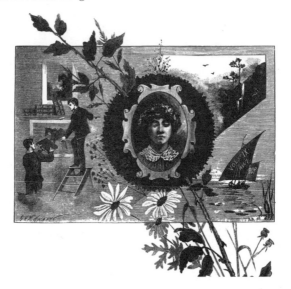

The Editor's attitude to girls in the *Answers to Correspondents* was more complex than straightforward sexism. In the answers that follow there is sometimes an acceptance that girls are more than 'just a pretty face', although the first answer I quote seems to suggest just that:

You will have learnt ere this by our award of prizes that we interpret the word 'readers' in the broadest way, and make sex no disqualification for the competitions. The paper is, of course, primarily intended for boys, but surely no lad would be so ungallant as to object to the stimulating rivalry of a pretty sister or cousin. [*Presumably, ugly sisters and cousins need not compete.*]

– oOo –

The passage appears in a book avowedly written for a party purpose; and as it is a question of the word of a spiteful woman against that of the Duke of Wellington and the majority of the nation, we prefer to think that the Iron Duke did not expose his troops to more dangers than necessary, and did win the battle of Waterloo on his merits. If it comes to mushrooms – dukes or otherwise – who was Lady Hamilton?

– oOo –

Mr. Hartley is the champion lawn-tennis player. We never heard of a lady champion.

– oOo –

MERMAID – Stay on shore. A ship is no place for girls to work. There is no such occupation, however, beyond the one you mention, and you would have to start something new.

– oOo –

We really do not know how to cure a young lady of saying 'Er'm, er'm' without hurting her feelings. We find it safer to leave the young ladies alone, and to devote all our attention to the boys. Er'm, er'm!

– oOo –

You need not apologise. We are always pleased to hear from girls as well as boys. Several letters express gratification at the permission for girls to join in the prize competitions of the BOY'S OWN PAPER until there is a 'Girl's Own

Paper' also. One lady, however, writing from Brighton, strongly objects to girls being encouraged to engage in literary work, as 'tending to increase the inordinate love of display and admiration, so repulsive in the present day.'

– oOo –

Any cookery-book will tell you how to make puff-paste. The question is one for the girls, not the boys. There is a solidity about the generality of boys' pastry efforts which is somewhat uninviting. They never do puff satisfactorily!

– oOo –

SIX DOZEN LADY READERS – There is no safe hair depilatory. Pray leave it alone. We do not want six dozen lady readers to have six dozen red faces, or twelve dozen red arms.

On one occasion, the BOY'S OWN PAPER was reprimanded by a reader's mother for what appeared to be a blatant insult to the female sex, and the Editor published the reprimand, only to turn the tables on the complainant and insult her in the process:

> A mother protests against the concluding words of the 26th chapter of 'Jack and John,' where the writer speaks of that 'useless, helpless thing – a woman.' She objects to boys being made to think thus of their mothers and sisters. This fond but dull mother does not see that the writer is speaking ironically and that stout Jenny was as useful to the 'poor helpless man' (Enoch) 'as if she were a good stout staff.'

Actually, when you read the paragraph complained of, in a story written by a woman, Mrs Eiloart, it's easy to see why 'A mother' was offended. The alleged irony is heavily concealed:

> Off Jim Dobbs drove with the boys, and as they turned to take a last look at Enoch and Jenny through the dull grey light of the early morning, they saw Jenny carefully leading Enoch back into the house, and he leaning on her as if she was a good stout staff instead of that worse than useless, helpless thing – a woman.

I suppose it was all seen as good clean knockabout fun, and at least the girls were sometimes allowed to have their say – about boys:

A GIRL'S OPINION OF THE BOYS – We have still very many girls of all ages amongst our admiring readers, as proved by the number of letters we receive from them. Amongst the latest is one that we thought it might interest the boys to see, so we give it *verbatim et literatim.* Perhaps they may have something to say in reply: – 'DEAR MR. EDITOR, – You know that lots of us girls read the "BOY'S OWN." I am not going to say which we like best – perhaps both; but what I wanted to say was, if we were boys, or boys were girls – I don't know which way to put it – after reading all that dreadful account of those poor slaves, just as Livingstone and Stanley wrote, knowing that it is all going on now, we should have got up committees and secretaries, and got petitions up to be signed by every reader of the "BOY'S OWN," and got some nice kind gentleman to take it to the House in a waggon, and make such a speech as would make those countries ashamed of themselves who encourage such wicked doings. But, there, boys never were of any use but to spin tops, pick out our dolls' eyes, rob birds' nests, tear their clothes, and make big holes in their stockings, and torment their sisters; that's the opinion of POLLY PEET.'

Only very rarely in *Answers to Correspondents* did sex – or at least love – rear its head. But boys, then as now, did occasionally fall in love with the irritating creatures and then had some difficulty knowing how to respond, or even whether the object of their affections returned the compliment:

If a young lady were to conclude a letter to us with 'and believe me to remain, yours truly,' we should in reply ask her to believe that we remained yours truly. In fact, there is no safer rule than to answer a letter in the terms and spirit in which it is written.

'Kind regards' is merely a polite formula, and when 'a young lady sends them to a young gentleman,' we would advise the young gentleman to assume that the young lady simply concluded her note in stereotyped phrase, and meant – nothing.

– o O o –

Fuzboz is mute; he can't advise. [*'Fusbos'* – *misspelt here* – *was a character in a burlesque opera, and the pen-name of a writer for* Punch.] Sympathy in such matters goes a long way; you have ours, and we give your case – alas! so typical – that you may receive that of our readers. Put the duel off, however, till you hear again – from us. 'I love a girl who is very pretty in my opinion, and another fellow wants to have her for his sweetheart, so I got cross with him, and he hit me, so I did not hit him back, and I shall duel with him either with butchers' knives or pistols. I consider myself quite worthy of her, for I wear a new-fashioned hat on Sunday, and a stick, and a flower, and black-and-white trousers, commonly called by cads pepper-and-salt.' Have you reflected that your hated rival perchance might spoil your pepper-and-salt?

– o O o –

If you are both of full age, there is no law to prevent you marrying your cousin – unless your cousin objects to marry you.

– o O o –

Had you looked at the Table of Affinity in your Prayer Book your anxiety would soon have ended. The marriage of cousins is not unlawful, but it is not desirable.

– o O o –

'Could you kindly tell me of a nice, inexpensive present to make my sweetheart!' What a question for an editor! Give her the seven volumes of the BOY'S OWN PAPER

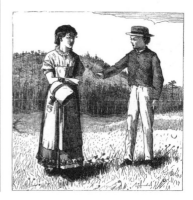

nicely bound in white vellum – and then tell her we recommended you to do so!

– oOo –

You are not the first that has been influenced by the moon. 'As I am very much in love with a young lady whose name is Diana, can you kindly inform me how I can gain her affections?' Well – keep your distance, and never say die. Tell her you have written to us for advice!

And even when troth was plighted, there were still vexing problems which it was hoped the B.O.P. could answer:

The fact of your being engaged to a lady should make no difference in the mark of respect that is due to her. You would, of course, raise your hat.

The other area where the B.O.P. slipped into what today would seem the height of political incorrectness was in matters of nationality and race. First, there was no doubt left in any reader's mind that the B.O.P. was British and proud of it, and that people of any other nationality, however civilized they might seem, were defective. Even though the story pages were full of tales of American pioneers and the Wild West, America and Americans were frequently singled out for disparagement – often gratuitously – in the *Correspondence* column:

BRITISHER and ANXIOUS INQUIRER are too much alike – in fact, 'the likeness between them is *sich* that we cannot tell either from both, and do not know t'other from which.' The 'splendid scholar, clever, tender-hearted, impulsive boy' of the one writes too much like the 'splendid speaker! remarkably clever! impulsive nature! young enough to learn any profession!' of the other, who is, however, 'rather lazy, but soon *shaked* off.' Such universal geniuses (if two of them do exist, and so modest and unassuming withal!) would be out of place in this old country. It is only in

America that such talents for self-advertisement would find a fitting field. Other correspondents please note.

– o O o –

... We cannot act on your advice to give coupons, lottery prizes and such things. These are schemes common in low-class journals in America. The object is obviously rather to push into circulation papers that cannot depend wholly upon their merits than to encourage wholesome and improving competition among boys.

– o O o –

U.S.A. MEDICAL DEGREE – Such a degree is no good here. There are so many bought or bogus ones.

– o O o –

We should say 'How do you do, sir?' and have no fear of the consequences. We should not address the official as 'Mr. Consul' or Mister anything. The use of the word Mister in such phrases, or by itself, is an Americanism, and on this side of the Atlantic is a vulgarism, which you would do well to avoid.

– o O o –

DUMPS – If you want to drop one of your Christian names, drop it, and say nothing and pay nothing. In legal documents you had better leave no doubt as to your identity; and, in the case of changing surname and paying for it, it is always best to describe yourself as, say, FitzFaddle, formerly Dumps. A lawyer would advise you. Why not Americanise your name, as, for instance, Ulysses Z. Dumps? 'Noblesse oblige' translates itself.

– o O o –

Avoid all such nostrums, and consult a properly qualified doctor. If you know the cause of an illness, cease the practice, or remove the cause, and then apply to a respectable medical man. Patent medicines are medicines that have, at the best, been found successful in a few instances, and are rashly assumed to be in consequence of value to all. But it by no means follows that they are so, and they are generally of more harm than good, especially in such cases as yours. You would hardly seek for absolute truth in such an American advertisement!

– o O o –

He is a Yankee quack. The very fact of his putting U.S. after his supposed title suggests that. The other firm is also that of a set of impudent quacks. Go to a doctor of course. Those who patronise advertising scoundrels deserve to suffer.

But the B.O.P. was unbiased in the foreigners it disliked:

Foreign readers of the BOY'S OWN PAPER are eligible for our competitions, but they must write in English, and take their chance – a poor one – with our British boys. The statement from Madame de Stael is the reverse of the truth. It is only in France that such things are invented and believed. The ship was captured by the English; the crew, instead of disappearing 'dans l'abîme,' went into Warwickshire.

– oOo –

We make no difference between Ireland and the rest of the kingdom. If anything good reaches us from Ireland we appreciated it, but you must excuse us from supposing that nothing but good can come out of your country. Be patriotic by all means, but such patriotism as yours can but make you ridiculous.

– oOo –

The greatest engineering work of the day is the Forth Bridge. The Eiffel Tower is mere child's play to it. Read our accounts of both, and judge for yourself.

– oOo –

VIKING – Indeed! What a misnomer! You have not a particle of our sympathy. You a viking, a descendant of the old sea kings, yet coolly averring that you 'intend emigrating to the States because the sea voyage is so much shorter than that to Australia!' An Englishman afraid of the sea! The expense argument we can understand, but – oh! you degenerate descendant of the men who gloried in riding out a North Sea gale in a boat the size of a fly-barge!

– oOo –

Thanks for your good opinion. For some wretched Swampville in Central Africa or South America the advice against early rising given in the cutting which you enclose may be all very well, though even those who live and work in India would tell you a very different tale. Ask our farmers or outdoor labourers in the colonies, no less than England, what they think of such nonsense, and they will laugh a laugh that will hardly suggest that the habit of following the lead of the sun has very seriously debilitated *them*.

– oOo –

The difference between an English and a German concertina is great. The English is usually an instrument of music, the German is an instrument of torture. The English is the original, the other the imitation. The English has forty-eight keys, the German twenty keys. Any good musical-instrument seller would supply you with one, but Wheatstone and Lachenal are supposed to be the best makers.

– oOo –

E. J. S. wishes to know 'whether tea-leaves are good for rabbits or not'. Neither good nor harm, in moderation; but tea-leaves are not British, and rabbits are best fed on the vegetables of their own country.

– oOo –

What next, we wonder. 'Is cricket of German origin?' Why, of course! All German; everything is of German origin – the sun, the moon, the universe, the BOY'S OWN PAPER – all German! 'Seek ye the Germ!'

Where late Victorian attitudes, as expressed in the BOY'S OWN PAPER, seem to us today really nasty is in matters of race. All races outside Europe and America were lumped together as an ignorant, violent and depraved mass, and sometimes legitimate targets for brave white men. This was expressed in many different ways in the stories and articles.

In *Queer Sport: A Barrister's Experiences in South Africa,* Hendrik B. Knoblauch described going Kafir-shooting:

> ... in a twinkling I fired, the bullet passing through him 'like a needle through sail cloth' ... To most Cape people, all blacks are <u>niggers</u>. It matters not whether they speak of the jet-black

Mozambiquer or of the bilious-looking Indian rajah. And they would as lief, in private life, associate with a monkey as with either of these or their connecting links; though as I have no hesitation in saying that, as a <u>servant</u>, the nigger is, in the majority of instances, far better treated at the Cape than is the English 'slavey' in her fatherland.

We get a more charitable view of 'Kafirs' from the Rev. Robin Matson, in his article *Kafir Lads:*

Great events are taking place in South Africa now. What about the people who live there? the native inhabitants of the land? the Kafirs? and what about Kafir lads? Such questions are often asked either in a tone or accompanied by some sign of contempt, or it may be at times of curiosity. As a man would feel curious of any other animals that lived there; and occasionally with a tone of patronage and pity as much as to say, 'Ah! what can we do for these inferior, these poor heathen?'

But you who read this are English lads, with young, free and generous hearts, not yet hardened by prejudices, and ready to own what is good and true and manly wherever you find it. Treat a Kafir as a fellow man and you will then know that the Kafirs are as fine a race as any made by God on this earth, and an example in some ways to many of us English, who mistakenly think and speak of the Kafirs as an inferior race.

The Kafir lads are a fine set of fellows – that's how I found them, and I simply could not help loving and admiring them ... I often think of them, their well-made figures and active rounded limbs [*steady there, Vicar*]; their innocent mirth and fun; their childlike simplicity, their anxiety and keenness to learn, and their complete trust. I know that some are otherwise, but it is too often because they have learned their vices from the white man, from so-called Christians.

But then there's a sting in the tail:

Mind, I speak of *Kafir* lads only. In South Africa, where I was for two years, there are many other races, as Hottentots and Damaras. Some of these are far inferior to the Kafir, but being nearly the same in colour are often confounded one with the other.

A universal target of opprobrium in stories and articles were American Indians, barbaric to a man:

A relic of Indian barbarism was received at the War Department at Washington recently. It consisted of a necklace of human fingers. Originally there were eleven fingers, strung together after the manner of necklaces of bears' claws, but three of them had been lost. This ghastly adornment was captured in an attack on the Northern Cheyennes in 1876, and each finger represented a life taken by the owner, the 'big medicine man' of the tribe. The fingers had been preserved by opening the skin, removing the bones, scraping away all the tissues and fatty substances, replacing the bones, and subjecting the skin to some tanning process. The necklace was sent to West Point by Captain Bourke, who is now engaged in preparing some historical matter relating to the Indians. It was brought from West Point in order that it might be reproduced in papier-mâché at the Smithsonian Institution.

For true ignorance, there is this 'comic' verse:

> There once was a funny old Sioux,
> Very partial to having a chew
> Of fresh Betel Nut,
> And enjoyed a prime cut
> Off a nicely baked captive or two.
> For he was a Cannibal bold
> While he had a sound tooth in his head.
> But when they wore out, I've been told,
> He seemed to prefer home made Bread.

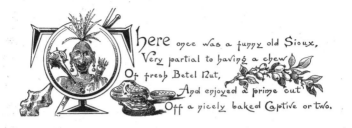

here once was a funny old Sioux,
Very partial to having a chew
Of fresh Betel Nut,
And enjoyed a prime cut
Off a nicely baked Captive or two.

This extraordinary piece of writing manages to confuse American Indians with Indian Indians (betel nuts) and ascribe to them a practice which is now seen as often mythical, or at least greatly exaggerated. But as a concession to truth, or half-truth, one answer to a correspondent gave a marginally less extreme account:

The Indians are nearly all half-civilised now, and the wandering tribes are few, it having been the endeavour of the Government to keep them as much has possible to 'Reservations' and the 'Indian Territory.

While apparently condemning the practices of some of these unspeakable people, the writers from B.O.P. knew that boys had an appetite for reading about them, which is why there were accounts like the following:

CANNIBALS – The black cannibals of Northern Queensland are reported as being partial to Chinamen. The reason is said to be that the flesh of the Chinese is peculiarly tender and palatable, owing to rice being their staple article of diet. There is now a numerous Chinese population in the north of Australia, and scores of them who have ventured beyond the confines of civilisation have been captured and devoured by the natives. This explains the nonchalance with which the Northern Queensland surveyor recently reported in these terms to the Government:– 'The blacks have stolen all my provisions and *sampled* two of my Chinamen.' 'Sampled' in this connection is rich indeed!

And this, from New Guinea:

> It was resting-day at a village, far away from the coast, and, spreading my chart out on the middle of the floor in the small native house in which we were camping, several sitting round, I was tracing our journey done and the probable one to do, when strange drops were falling around, a few on the chart. They came from a bulky parcel overhead. Jumping up quickly, I discovered that they were grandmother's remains being dried. Our chart was placed on the fire, and the owner was called lustily, who hurriedly entered and walked away with the parcel. This horrible way of treating the dead is curious enough, but it is by no means the most curious thing in the new book on New Guinea just issued by the Religious Tract Society ...

'Natives' were generally treated as physically and mentally inferior. Replies in *Answers to Correspondents* emphasised the smaller brain size of non-British people:

According to Morton, the Englishman has the largest brain-case. Next to him comes the German and Anglo-American. The Irishman comes next to the Malay.

– oOo –

The highest brain capacity of the European at present known is 114 cubic inches; the brain capacity of the lowest Hindu is only 46 cubic inches. There is a difference, therefore, of 68 cubic inches between the highest and the lowest. But the highest brain capacity of the gorilla yet measured is 34^1/$_2$ inches. There is thus less difference between the gorilla and the lowest Hindu than there is between the lowest Hindu and the highest European.

– oOo –

In the typical negro there is a great difference shown. The arm is two inches longer in proportion than that of a Caucasian, and the hands hang level with the kneecaps; the facial angle is 70 as against 83; the brain weighs 35 as against 45; the skull is much thicker; the heel projects backwards; the great toe is feebly prehensile; the frame is not upright; and there is no growth in intelligence once manhood is reached.

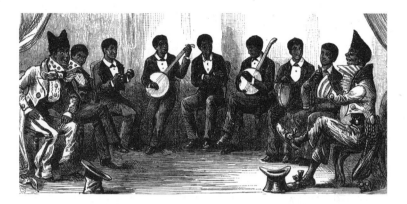

However, there was one particular, more benign, reference to black people which appeared time and again in the columns of the B.O.P. which referred to the presence in Victorian popular culture of 'Nigger minstrels' – usually, in fact, white people with blackened faces who sang and danced, and played the 'bones':

Burnt cork is the best thing for nigger entertainments. Make it yourself.

– oOo –

We do not know of a guide to 'the bones,' nor of any music specially written for that instrument. The great secret is to waggle them furiously, and make as much noise as you can. The 'blacking' is simply powdered burnt cork.

– oOo –

Prepared burnt cork is sold by many music-sellers for blacking the face at nigger entertainments. The time taken to wash it off depends very much on your skin and the way you wash.

Reflecting the enthusiasm for 'nigger minstrels', there was an article about 'The American Dancing Nigger.'

It is now some years since one evening at Christmas time I made one of a large family party assembled at the house of a relation. The evening had passed very pleasantly, and we were chatting

THE AMERICAN DANCING NIGGER.

By C. Stansfeld-Hicks.

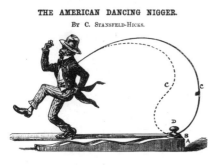

together, and watching an arrangement which was being made in a recess behind a pair of curtains, before which was a small table. After some little time waiting in expectation, there suddenly appeared from between the curtains the agile gentleman who is portrayed at the head of this article. The operator, concealed (all but a portion of his arm) behind the curtains, placing the stand on the table, and cleverly manipulating the wire, caused the figure to dance in the most amusing and ridiculous manner, creating the greatest merriment. Afterwards, some lively jigs and reels being played on the piano, the figure footed it away, cleverly keeping time to the music.

Coming across the stand of the figure brought the memory of it to my mind, and I thought that making and working such a figure would be an amusing occupation for some of the readers of the BOY'S OWN PAPER in the long winter evenings.

The nigger, when he first came out, was rather an expensive toy, and I have not latterly seen anything quite like it, but it is within the capabilities of any ingenious lad to make one for himself at a very small expense. The one I have described was about eight inches high, and had a proportionately sized stand; but of course it can be made of any size, though a smaller one would be quite as troublesome to make, and not so funny. We will take the figure as being about the height described ...

For boys, many of them, who might seek a career in the colonies, the B.O.P. with its unthinking reflections on 'foreigners' was not a particularly useful guide to the people they would be likely to meet.

WORDS AND PHRASES

ENTIRE

'Entire' on a public-house sign means simply 'porter.' Originally three different sorts of beer were mixed to give the taste of porter; then a man succeeded in brewing a beer combining the characteristics of the three, which was in consequence called 'Entire;' which 'Entire,' as being a drink much approved of by porters and the rougher classes, eventually became known as 'Porter.'

REMEMBER THE GROTTO

'Please remember the grotto!' is a reminder not to forget your offering to St. James the Great, on whose day the request is made. It used to be the custom on the day to stick a shell in your hat or cloak, and pay a visit to the shrine of St. James of Compostella; and, for the benefit of those who could not afford the pilgrimage, shell grottoes were erected with the image of the saint to serve the same purpose. The saint's image has given place to the humble tallow candle, or, rather, the light has remained and the image has gone; and the custom has degenerated into an excuse for the extraction of halfpennies on the part of small boys who know nothing of the serious nature of the early grottoes, and look upon them as started for the sole purpose of announcing that the 'oyster season has now commenced.'

PEPPER GATE

'When your daughter is stolen close Pepper Gate' is equivalent to 'When your horse is stolen lock the stable door.' Pepper Gate is at Chester, and when the mayor's daughter eloped through it, the mayor, wise man! ordered the gate to be locked, lest some other daughter should do likewise.

CARNIVAL

Carnival means 'good-bye, meat,' and is the last full-dinner feast for six weeks. Hence all the jollification attempted to be squeezed into it for which the following fast is to atone. It was of gradual growth, and is a survival of one of the many old Roman festivities which seem to have been numerous enough to have originated every holiday now kept in Europe.

HATS

A wideawake hat is a hat that never sleeps – in fact, one that never has, or had, a *nap*. All felts are napless. Jim Crow hats were so called from being worn by that famous nigger minstrel. Beaver hats were made of beaver skins. The Billy-cock hat was invented by a Mr. Wilcock, facetiously familiarised into Mr. Billycock.

HARVEST MOON

For about a week during the time that the harvest moon is at the full there is very little difference between the time of her rising on any two successive nights, the reason being that her orbit is then nearly parallel with the horizon. The same thing occurs in the spring, but then the moon is not full at the time, and it is therefore not so noticeable.

HOOKEY WALKER

Hookey Walker, so called from his beaked nose, was a clerk in Cheapside, and his duties were to supervise the workmen. His reports were discredited, and hence 'Hookey Walker!' came to be a slang expression for 'I don't believe it!' This is the explanation usually given, but the reply to it is generally 'Hookey Walker!'

JACK ROBINSON

We do not know who the original Jack Robinson was, but Mr. Halliwell cites an old play in which the saying appears as 'as easie to be done as tys to say Jacke! robys on.'

SET THE THAMES ON FIRE

To set the Thames on fire is to do something startling in the world. It is an old pun with the joke gone – as usual. The temse – not the Thames – was the corn sieve which was worked over the sifted flour. A hardworking man would occasionally work the siftings so energetically as to set fire to the wooden hoop at the bottom. Hence the sluggard would never set the temse on fire with the grain. We are loth to add that this derivation is usually taken *cum grano*.

UNIVERSAL SACK

There is one word whose sound is said to have the same meaning in all languages, and that is 'sack' in the sense of a bag.

LIKE A TOP

When a top is spinning so fast and steadily that it does not seem to move, it is said to sleep. Hence 'sleep like a top.'

CHESHIRE CAT

Cheese in Cheshire (and, by-the-by, Cheshire is not Cheese-shire, although it looks as if it ought to be) was occasionally made up into fancy shapes, much as butter is now, and one of the shapes was that of a cat with a most interesting smile. Hence people who show much of their teeth when they laugh are often rudely said 'to grin like a Cheshire cat.'

DINING WITH DUKE HUMPHREY

Humphrey, Duke of Gloucester, uncle of Henry VII, was renowned for his hospitality. When he died it was reported that a monument was to be erected to him in St. Paul's, but he was buried at St. Albans; and for many years afterwards, when the strollers in St. Paul's left to go to dinner, those who remained behind used to say that they were not going home yet, but would stay a little longer, and look for the monument of the 'good duke.' Hence 'dining with Duke Humphrey' was dining on nothing.

PLOUGH MONDAY

It was so called from being the first Monday after the Christmas holidays, after which the men returned to work. Before doing so they used to draw a plough from door to door through the parish, and ask for alms towards a final carouse.

CHRISTMAS BOXES

Christmas boxes probably owe their origin to a primitive methods of taking the census! In the old days of Rome, as far back as the time of the mythical Servius Tullius, an altar was erected in every village about the time of our present Christmas, and on it each man, woman, or child residing in the district had to drop a single coin, its value being immaterial. The coins, being counted, gave the numbers of the population; and the amount so subscribed was distributed to the most deserving. The custom lived on: census-papers took the place of counters, pockets took the place of altars; the alteration of the faith made no alteration in the seasonable custom, and it gradually became modified as we now have it.

CATS AND DOGS

The meaning of 'raining cats and dogs'? It means raining heavily. The origin is simple. The catkins of poplar and the willow are very fluffy, and in some districts are known as 'pussies' and 'pups.' On the trees they are hardly noticed, but when the heavy rain comes it brings them down, and it was thought at one time to bring them with it from the clouds. The phrase is thus due to the descent of the catkin, or little cat, or little puss, or pussie, swept off by a shower! This is the recognised derivation unless you prefer the 'catadoupe' or waterfall of the French; or share the opinion of the sceptics, who see no more meaning in it than in 'raining like old boots,' and ascribe both phrases to a common origin, a mere jingle invented in a hurry by some unknown in a futile attempt to say something smart.

BRICK TALK

When you say that a fellow is a brick, it is the slang for an honest upright lad, though that depends on the person using the word. A scamp would probably think another scamp a 'brick' if ready to act along with him. The origin of the phrase may be this: bricks are made of a certain size or shape, nine inches long, four and a half wide, and three thick. Hence build bricks whatever way you please, lengthways, edgeways, or flat, they will always build true and square. Some persons, however, assert that the expression is of classical origin. A nobler phrase is that used by Tennyson when he describes the great Duke of Wellington as 'four-square to all the winds that blow.' 'Acting on the square' is also used to denote straightforward honourable conduct. If W. [the questioner] is tired of calling a good fellow a 'brick,' he may call him 'a cube,' which is always true, and the slang would have a reason and right meaning for it. An honest fellow or a truthful boy, would give a higher and better idea of character than such slang as 'brick' which has bad as well as good applications.

BEANFEAST

The beanfeast is said to be a north-country term for the goose-feast, the bean-goose coming next in size to the grey-lag. It is thus akin to wayz-goose – the goose dinner eaten in common by the workmen of a firm once a year. It is also said to come from the cake with a bean in it, which conferred the presidency of the feast, on Twelfth Night principles, to the happy possessor of the slice with the bean in it.

CARSHALTON

Names ending in 'halton,' like those ending in 'ham,' do not have the 'sh' sound. The pronunciation is Cars Halton, and the Cars is abbreviated first into Cays, then into Kers, and so on, until you get the Ksalton of the railway-porters.

GORDIAN KNOT

The Phrygians wanted a new king, and the Oracle told them to choose the first man they met going to the temple of Jupiter on a chariot. This turned out to be Gordius, who immediately dedicated his chariot to Jupiter, and tied the pole up to a beam in a knot of such a pronounced 'granny's' type that neither he nor anyone else could undo it. At length it became a saying that he who could untie this knot would secure the empire of the East; and consequently Alexander the Great, in his passage across Asia Minor, called in at Gordium, and finding the knot a teaser, promptly cut it with his sword.

CRUDEN'S SPONGE

We never met with the phrase, 'Cruden's Sponge,' before, but suppose it is an allusion to the sponge which Alexander Cruden used to carry about with him, and with which he used to wipe out all the objectionable words and drawings with which rude boys had ornamented the walls and palings of his native town.

LETTERS AND NUMBERS

ROMAN NUMERALS

The fact that M of the Roman notation is the initial letter of mille – the word meaning a thousand – is simply a coincidence, just as it is that C is the initial of centum, a hundred. The first system of the Romans consisted entirely of vertical strokes, and, in order to facilitate the counting of these, they were divided into groups of ten each by two lines crossing them diagonally. (Very much the same sort of thing is seen on modern wine-casks to note the gallons removed.) After a time the cross began to stand alone without the vertical strokes it cancelled, and these St. Andrew's crosses at last became X's. These X's were afterwards marked off into groups of ten by similar cancelling, consisting in this case of two parallel horizontal lines drawn through them, and joined by a vertical line at the end. This rectangular figure afterwards stood alone, just as the X had become to do, and at last was shortened and rounded off into the C. Then, to save the five separate strokes, the X was cut into half, and its upper half did for the V; and then, to save marking the five X's, the rectangular C was cut in half, and the lower part became the L. Then the C and the V, in their rectangular forms, were combined, and the result was the D, and then the C was crossed and became the M. Then, for the IIII, IV, meaning 1 from 5, was adopted; and for the VIIII, IX, meaning 1 from 10, and so on. In later times the notation was extended to , representing 10,000, , representing 100,000, and these were halved. The Romans had no arithmetic to speak of, they used the Abacus. If you want a little excitement, work out a cube root with the Roman notation.

COINCIDENCES

On 5 December 1664, a boat was crossing the Menai Straits, when it upset, and out of eighty-one persons only one was saved. His name was Hugh Williams. On 5 December 1785, another boat was crossing the Menai Straits, when it upset, and out of sixty passengers only one was saved. His name was Hugh Williams! On 5 August 1820, another boat was crossing the Menai Straits, when it upset, and out of twenty-five persons only one was saved. His name was Hugh Williams!

Coincidences are endless – and worthless. You cannot think about anything without finding coincidences of some sort. Take Louis XIV, for example. He was born in 1643, and 1+6+4+3=14; he died in 1715, and 1+7+1+5=14; and he was 77 years old, and 7+7=14. Take Louis Philippe, who was crowned in 1830; he was born in 1773, and 1830+1+7+7+3=1848, when, as 'Mr. Smith,' he appeared in a hurry at Newhaven; his queen was born in 1782, and 1830+1+7+8+2=1848; and he had fled in 1809, and 1830+1+8+0+9=1848. An ingenious mind will find coincidences in everything, from Pyramids to Pantomimes. Napoleon III was crowned in 1852; he was born in 1808, and 1852+1+8+0+8=1869, his last year of success. Eugenie was born in 1826, and 1808+1+8+2+6=1869. Or, to crown all, take his uncle, Napoleon I, of whom it was discovered that 'Napoleon Apollyon is a lion going about destroying cities,' inasmuch as if you gradually decapitate him you get 'Napoleon – apoleon – poleon – oleon- leon – eon!

UNIVERSITY COSTS

It costs an average student at Oxford or Cambridge close on £300 in fees, board, lodging, and expenses, before he takes his B.A. degree. 2. At Keble College, Oxford, there is an annual charge of £82 to cover rent, board, tuition, and all necessary expenses except washing, light, and drink. 3. At Corpus Christi, Cambridge, the charges are £2 per quarter for bedmaker, £1 13s. 4d. for coals, £1 1s. 6d. for boots, £1 15s. for laundress, from

£3 10s. to £8 10s. for rent, etc., £15 for steward, and £6 for tuition.

DESCENDANTS

We are delighted to hear that we have just the 1/8589934592nd part of our ancestor of a thousand years ago, but we are in no way comforted or appalled thereby. We have no doubt he was an exceedingly good fellow, and so were all the other 8,589,934,591 to whom you assure us we are indebted. As, however, the world is pretty full now, and it has only 1,400,000,000 inhabitants, we fail to see for the moment how it managed to contain half a dozen times as many in the days of King Alfred. However, there is nothing like statistics. We should not wonder if one of the 8,589,934,592 was not some relation of yours; and so, as a presumably distant cousin, we quite agree with you.

EQUATION OF PAYMENTS

The rule by which you tell the approximate due date of two or more amounts due at different dates is known as 'Equation of Payments.' The mode is to multiply each debt by the time that must elapse before it will become due, and then divide the sum of the products thus obtained by the sum of the debts to get the time required; or else to multiply each debt except the one that is payable earliest, by the difference between its time and the time for that one, and then divide the sum of the products by the sum of the debts, and add the quotient to the time for the first debt. Take the time in days.

GENERATIONS

A generation is the interval of time that elapses between the birth of a father and the birth of his son – or, in other words, the number of years that persons are on the average younger than their fathers or mothers. As far back as the days of Herodotus this was observed to average thirty-three years and four months, or three generations to each century, and it is still taken as such. With the Stuart Kings of Scotland it was curiously enough true to a day. From observations on the population of Paris made in 1829, the period was found to be 33.31 years; and in 1874 a new inquiry into our own population statistics gave us 34.48. No less than five generations have been known to be living in one family, hence the stanza:

> The aged mother to her daughter spake -
> 'Daughter,' said she, 'arise,
> Thy daughter to her daughter take,
> Whose daughter's daughter cries.

REMEMBERING MORSE

Of course the code requires practice, but what so many have done you ought to do. It may help you to know that certain words can be found beginning with the letter sought having the same number of syllables as the signal has dots and dashes, and having its longs and shorts in the same order. For instance, A is made by a dot and a dash, and can be remembered by About. Barbarously can stand for B, its syllables consisting of a long and three shorts. Calculator will do for C, a long and short and long and short. Dreamily will do for D, a long and two shorts. Et will do for E, one short. Filibuster will do for F, two dots, a dash, and a dot. Golconda will do for G, two longs and a dot. Hurry-hurry will do for the four shorts of H. Ibi will do for the two shorts of I. Judiciousness will do for the short and three longs of J. Kitchen-maid for the long, short, long of K. Lamellarly for the short, long, two shorts of L. Mousetrap for the two longs of M. Noodle for the long and short of N. Oh! oh! oh! for the three longs of O. Provokingly for the short, long, long, short of P.

Queen's Head Hotel for the long, long, short, long of Q. Reviler for the short, long, short of R. Similar for the three shorts of S. Tape for the one long of T. Unabridged for the two shorts and a long of U. Very remote for the three shorts and a long of V. Whereunto for the short and two longs of W. Xanthidium for the long, short, short, long of X. Yesternight week for the long, short, long, long of Y; and Zoology for the long, long, two shorts of Z.

PRINTER'S PIE

Hardly any occupation exists of which startling statistics could not be compiled. Even a compositor setting type has been reckoned up, and it appears that one Michael Quin, of the Erie 'Daily Herald,' has handled 358,020,000 pieces of metal twice over, that the metal so lifted would weigh ninety-four tons, and that in setting it in position his hand has travelled 516,000,000 feet, or 97,727 miles, or nearly four times the circumference of the globe!

TAKE A LETTER

The letterer's scale for sign-painting is as follows. Supposing the height of the capital letters to be ten inches, then the widths of B, F, and P will be ten inches, of A C D E G H K N O Q R T V X and Y eleven inches, of I five inches, of J eight inches, of S and L nine inches, of M and W seventeen inches, and of Z and & twelve inches. If the lower-case letters are thirteen inches high, then a b d k p x and z will be fifteen inches wide, c e o and s fourteen inches, f i j l and t six inches, g h n and u sixteen inches, m twenty-six inches, r v and y twelve inches, and w twenty inches.

SQUARES MADE EASY

There is a way of squaring numbers by complement and supplement, if that is what you mean by the American system. We first met with it in a little work called 'Lightning Arithmetic,' published in San Francisco by G. Frusher Howard. You take the ten next before the number, add to the number to be squared the difference between it and the ten, multiply that by the ten, and then square the difference you got at first and add it to the result. Thus to square 13 you take the nearest ten behind it, which happens to be 10, subtract it from 13, and get 3; then you add 3 to 13, and multiply by 10 – in other words, 13+3x10=160; and then you add the square of 3, namely, 9, so that the full calculation runs (13+3x10)+9=169. In large numbers the gain is great, thus – 1007 squared=(1007+7x1000)+49, or 1,014,049. This is called squaring by supplement; squaring by complement is taking the ten next in front of the number, and subtracting instead of adding. Thus 993 squared would be (993-7x1000)+49=986.

THE NUMBER 13

The superstitious notion that if thirteen sit down to table a death is sure to occur is due to the fact that at the Last Supper there were thirteen persons. If that number sit at a meal it is quite true that one will die eventually – so will all, in fact; and so will they all if more or less than thirteen partake of the meal. The thing is of course ridiculous, though it has just that spice of half-truth which keeps it alive.

MOLECULES

Mr. Sorby has calculated that in every cubic thousandth of an inch of water the molecules number 3,700,000,000,000,000 – three thousand seven hundred million millions, or, if you like it better, three thousand seven hundred billions. Count as fast as you can you will never count more than a quarter of a million a day.

SEVENS

SEVEN SLEEPERS OF EPHESUS

The seven Sleepers of Ephesus were seven young men who fled to a cave in Mount Celion during the persecution of the Christians under Decius, and there fell asleep. The mouth of the cave was stopped up, but they continued in peaceful slumber for two hundred and thirty or three hundred and nine years, according to which legend you prefer. They then awoke, but lived for only a short time. Their dog Katmir followed them into the grave, but they threw stones at him to drive him away, and even broke three of his legs. The dog, however, refused to move, and at last found speech to say, 'I love those who love God. Sleep, masters, and I will keep guard.' Which he did until his masters awoke. During their long sleep the youths turned frequently on their sides, and every time they did so some great disaster occurred to the faith. The bones of the sleepers were taken to Marseilles.

SEVEN WISE MEN OF GREECE

The Seven Wise Men of Greece and their favourite maxims were: 1. Solon of Athens – 'Know thyself.' 2. Chilo of Sparta – 'Consider the end.' 3. Thales of Miletus – 'Who hateth suretyship is sure.' 4. Bias of Priene – 'Most men are bad.' 5. Cleobulos of Lindos – 'Avoid extremes.' 6. Pittacos of Mitylene – 'Seize time by the forelock.' 7. Periander of Corinth – 'Nothing is impossible to industry.'

SEVEN WONDERS

The seven wonders of the world were – The Pyramids of Egypt, the Mausoleum of Artemisia, the Temple of Diana at Ephesus, the Hanging Gardens of Babylon, the Colossus of Rhodes, the

Statue of Jupiter Olympus by Phidias, and the Pharos, or Watch Tower, of Alexandria. Nearly everything since achieved in the engineering or architectural way has been called the eighth wonder; but the term for a very long period was applied to the Escurial in Spain, which was built by Philip II to commemorate his victory over the French at St. Quentin. It was dedicated to St. Lawrence, and the saint's gridiron served as the model of the ground-plan, the architect, Juan Battista de Toledo, ingeniously making the bars out of lines of buildings, and the handle out of a church! It is nearly a mile round, and was built on the site of some old ironworks. Somebody once took the trouble to take stock of it, and found 1,860 rooms, 6,200 doors and windows, 80 staircases, 73 fountains, 48 wine-cellars, 51 bells, and 8 organs. It is the biggest and dreariest palace that ever was built.

SEVEN WONDERS IN VERSE

Better have them, then, in Dr. Brewer's version:-

> The Pyramids first which in Egypt were laid,
> Then Babylon's Garden for Amytis made,
> Then Mansolo's tomb of affection and guilt,
> Then the temple of Dian in Ephesus built,
> The Colossus of Rhodes, cast in brass, to the sun,
> Sixth Jupiter's statue by Phidias done,
> The Pharos of Egypt last wonder of old,
> Or the Palace of Cyrus cemented with gold.

SEVEN MORE WONDERS

The Seven Wonders of the World? Yes. Here they are – the very latest – all in the same delivery. Wonder 1 is CONSTANT READER, who has 'read the paper right through from the beginning, and could not possibly have missed them.' Wonder 2, A READER OF THE 'BOY'S OWN PAPER' who 'does not understand an index and believes that his 'nom de plum' will prevent his mistaking anybody else's answer' for his own. Wonder 3, W.M. per R.J.W. who wants the wonders 'primeval, midevial, and modern.' Wonder 4, AN OLD BOY, who 'has admired the BOY'S OWN PAPER for the last twenty years.' Wonder 5, F. NORMAN, who wonders why he never gets an answer, and concludes his letter with 'this is the first time I have troubled you.' Wonder 6, J., who expects us to show him the 'invisable motto on a penny.' Wonder 7, B.O.P. who, 'assisted by his uncle, looked all through the hundred and tenth number' and failed to find the Seven Wonders in the second Correspondence column. There are many other wonders but this time we draw the line at seven.

EPITAPHS

WATCHMAKER

There is a curious epitaph at Lydford, in Devon, on a watchmaker's tomb, which may be that referred to. It is stated to be as follows: –

> Here lies in a horizontal position
> the outside case of
> GEORGE ROUTLEDGE, Watchmaker.
> Integrity was the mainspring,
> and prudence the regulator, of all the actions of his life;
> Humane, generous, and liberal,
> His hand never stopped till he had relieved distress.
> So nicely regulated were his movements that he never went wrong,
> Except when set agoing by people who did not know his key:
> Even then he was easily set right again.
> He had the art of disposing of his time so well,

That his hours glided away in one continued round of pleasure,
Till in an unlucky moment his pulse stopped beating.
He ran down Nov. 14, 1801, aged 57,
In hopes of being taken in hand by his Maker,
Thoroughly cleaned, repaired, wound up, and set agoing
In the world to come, when time shall be no more.

SURVEYOR

The epitaph is probably the one at Enfield on a monument to John White, Surveyor to the New River Company from Lady Day, 1691, to Midsummer, 1723 – evidently on a quarterly engagement. The epitaph runs:

> Here lies John White, who day by day
> On river works did use much clay,
> Is now himself turning that way.
> If not to clay yet dust will come,
> Which to preserve takes little room,
> Although enclosed in this great tomb.

Chapter 5

'BETTER BE A PROSPEROUS MECHANIC THAN A NEEDY CLERK'

Jobs for the Boys

THE age range of B.O.P. readers was very wide. Setting aside the occasional letter from a surgeon – 'I see the Boy's Own Paper every month and read it with much interest' – or military officer, the ages of regular readers probably ran from ten or eleven to the early twenties. And a preoccupation for some of the 'boys' in the upper age range was the topic of a career. What were they going to do for a living – for those who needed to make a living?

It's in this area that the B.O.P.'s ideas on class came to the fore. The magazine tried to answer queries about the sort of jobs that would or wouldn't do for particular boys from a reasonably liberal standpoint:

The fact of being the son of a tradesman is no legal disqualification for holding a commission, whether in the Royal Artillery or the Royal Engineers.

– oOo –

You say you are a poor working man's son, but we are just as particular in answering queries from the cottage as from the castle.

– oOo –

We do not recognise any classes in this paper – working or otherwise. We cater for all. For us all boys are equal; we know them only as readers.

– oOo –

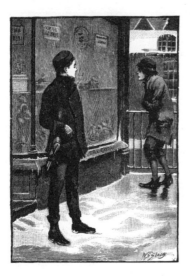

The volunteer service is 'below' no lad, however exalted he may be – in his own esteem or any one else's; and we should indeed despair of our country if such miserable snobbery were ever to prevail in any of our counties. Hold up your head, 'Volunteer,' and let us think more favourably of our friends! None but a noodle would harbour such an unworthy thought.

– oOo –

We are as pleased to advise a poor lad as a prince.

Boys' queries about Careers ranged from the general to the very specific:

ONE ANXIOUS FOR WORK – As 'any sedentary occupation knocks you up' and you are 'unfitted for outdoor occupation' we can scarcely advise you in the choice of a profession. Have you not, unconsciously perhaps, exaggerated your ailments?

– oOo –

Large game hunting is rarely pursued for profit. If you are successful enough, of course it would pay; but it would take a good many elephants and lions and so on to repay the money spent on such an expedition if you intend going single-handed. Your question is too vague. The expedition might cost you a thousand pounds.

– oOo –

It rests with the examining doctor; if he thinks that the candidate's teeth are not in a fit state for chewing biscuit he will not accept him.

– oOo –

In all questions about shorthand apply to Mr. Pitman, Paternoster Row, whom we really cannot go on advertising at this rate; so all readers contemplating queries on the subject, please note.

– o O o –

We should advise you to stay at home and work assiduously at your business. Did you ever hear of the dog and shadow? There is more truth in that old fable than young enterprising folks imagine. It is not so easy as you think to make a 'good position in the world,' and when you have one ready made your safest course would be to stick to it, and make your further efforts from that standpoint. There is a far nobler philosophy of life, however, than the 'get money, honestly, my lad, if you can, but get money.'

– o O o –

Our advice in the matter would simply be 'don't,' especially as you offer no evidence that you have any special talents in that direction.

– o O o –

Student interpreters proceed to Constantinople as soon as possible after passing their examination, where they are placed under the orders of the British Ambassador, for the purpose of studying Turkish, Persian, Slav, and Mohammedan law. The salary is £200 a year for five years, together with lodgings and tutors. A student interpreter must execute a bond for £500, which is forfeited should he leave or be dismissed for incompetence or bad conduct before the expiration of the five years. The age is 18 to 25, and a candidate must be a British subject, physically fit, and unmarried. The examination consists of (obligatory) arithmetic to decimal fractions, dictation, English composition, French, Latin; and (optional) Greek, Italian, German, Spanish. The competition is open, and advertised in the 'Times.' The examination fee is £4. A student interpreter *may* become a consul-general, at a salary of £2,000 a year.

– o O o –

Work hard and continuously, and you will succeed; but if you abandon any subject, let it be higher mathematics ...

– o O o –

We cannot undertake to advise any one as to what trade or profession he should choose. It is extremely unlikely that we should ever be thoroughly acquainted with all the circumstances of any individual case, and unless these are taken into consideration, advice would be misleading. You must choose for yourself. As a general rule, the man with special knowledge is the man who gets on. The future of the modern clerk, as a clerk and nothing more, seems to us very gloomy. There is a phantom gentility after which some people strive which is the cause of a vast deal of misery. Better be a prosperous mechanic than a needy clerk.

– oOo –

You had far better stay at home until you have learnt more about the United States. The idea of buying a farm, and making a living by 'going out shooting,' is merely a boyish dream, and we do not think any part of America would be suitable 'for that sort of thing.' If you think of emigrating, study the country you are going to, and fit yourself as well as you can for your new position.

– oOo –

There is no examination for the post of Home Secretary, etc. The position is not open to public competition –

at any rate by way of Cannon Row. You can get all information from the Civil Service Commissioners on application at their offices, but it is perfectly hopeless for you to think of getting into the service without passing an examination.

– oOo –

Never go to sea on a month's trial. You are sure to be disgusted. Boys are always ill during the first month. Go on a long voyage if you want to have a fair idea of what a seafaring life is like.

– oOo –

The good of it? Did you ever hear the story of Euclid and the boy? The boy, after learning the first proposition, asked what was the use of it. 'Here,' said Euclid, 'give the boy threepence, since he must make money out of everything he learns.' If you are to conduct your education solely with a view to making money by it your plans are not unlikely to miscarry.

– oOo –

A slight stammering would be no disqualification for the post unless there were many applicants. Of course, if it comes to choosing between two men otherwise equal, the non-stammerer would be chosen.

– o O o –

Your idea of making your living by hunting, either in the Himalayas or Rockies, is quite impracticable. There is no such book on the Himalayas. A good hunting-book on the Rocky Mountains is Mr. Baillie-Grohman's 'Camps in the Rockies,' published by Sampson Low and Co.

– o O o –

There is little use in your going to South America unless you can speak Spanish. When you have learnt that language an advertisement would almost certainly procure you a situation for a short term, which would give you a chance of visiting the country. Say nothing about your private income.

– o O o –

A CONSTANT PERUSER – You should 'peruse' a little less. You might then notice more, for your questions have been frequently answered. Men promoted from the ranks have to pass a certain educational examination in addition to their technical examination. No man can be promoted without an educational certificate. Men who cannot read or write are never anything else than privates.

– o O o –

All other things being equal, a tall man would always be chosen in preference to a short one; and you had much better stay where you are. Your handwriting is very good, but much too large and bold for a book-keeper. The firm that employed you would require such broad pages and wide lines that it would cost them a fortune in stationery.

– o O o –

You might work your passage out as an under-steward, but it would be better to have introductions to some one in China before you start. For one success we hear of so many failures that we decline to advise. If you are the right man for the place, you will do; if you are not, you will not.

– o O o –

For a situation as cook's boy apply to the captain of the ship or the secretary of the steamship company; but in making the application do not write on gilt-edged paper.

– o O o –

A. B. C. – The fate of the page-boy who is getting fatter than his master likes is indeed unenviable. Unless you turn over a new leaf your master will get a fresh page, and then what will you do? Hard lines on the page, and, as you hint, little justification! Eat less bread and potatoes, and take more exercise, O alphabetical buttons! and as a page you are bound to remain.

– oOo –

EMPLOYMENT FOR BOY (Anxious mother) – If so fond of natural history, why not try nursery gardening, as the lad is not strong enough for farming? He is not thriving, so cannot be too much out of doors. The sea will hardly do. Meanwhile he must not over-study, and should take good food and cod-liver oil.

– oOo –

LUMP ON NECK – Yes, it will stop you from entering either service if it is a glandular swelling.

– oOo –

It is hopeless your trying for a situation under Government unless you are healthy in all respects. The competition is so keen that even a defect in the teeth might cause your rejection.

– oOo –

So very much depends upon the natural bent of your own mind, and the influence your family might be able to exert in your favour, that we really could not undertake to say what trade or profession would be the best for you. Carey did not make a particularly good shoemaker, but what a fine linguist and glorious missionary he became! Many, on the other hand, fail utterly in professions, who at mechanical trades might have done well. Confer with your friends.

– oOo –

We have no means of knowing your likes and dislikes. As a rule, seventeen is too old to go to sea.

– oOo –

Many of the younger boys wrote in with queries about their apprenticeships. By working long hours for little or no pay in an occupation they hoped to take up, they would learn their craft – if they were under a good master. But here, the B.O.P. was surprisingly illiberal. Having given the impression in other areas that it stood up for the rights of 'our boys', in this case, where there was a choice between the rights of the apprentice and those of the master, the B.O.P. usually came down heavily on the side of the master.

We never answer legal questions. Our advice to ill-treated apprentices invariably has been 'to grin and bear it.' In many cases there are faults on both sides, and at the worst the tyranny will end at a stated time. Do your best, learn all you can; and when in due time it comes to you to be a master, think of what you have suffered as a warning, and do not ill-treat the poor lads that are then entrusted to you.

– oOo –

IGNORAMUS – like other apprentices who are constantly writing to us, should do all he can to please his master and learn his trade, and make light of any hardships or inconveniences he may have to put up with. The more work, and the greater variety of work, he has to do, the better for his future career. His master should be his friend, not his enemy, and he would be better engaged in assisting him in every way than in worrying himself as to the legality or advisability of such petty matters.

– oOo –

An apprentice should do whatever he is told, however irksome it may be. There is no law that draws the line between what is and what is not necessary for him to learn. Let him learn to obey – and keep his eyes open.

– oOo –

L. J. A. writes to know whether an apprentice who should run away and join the army or navy could be brought back. We think the best and kindest reply to such a question is simply, Don't think of trying it. Both honour and happiness usually come only in the path of duty; and running away from one's legitimate obligations is a poor, mean way of beginning the battle of life.

– oOo –

Such petty tricks are played in all trades. Do as your master bids you; and, when you are out of your time, remember the lesson, and do not put your own apprentices in a similar difficulty.

– o O o –

Fifteen hours a day is, we consider, much too long for a boy of fourteen to have to work; but we do not see what you can do except complete your apprenticeship. You should not have chosen a trade in which such long hours are customary.

– o O o –

We regret that your master's wife orders you to do things 'in an austere manner' without your master's permission; but your best plan is to grin and bear it. P.S. – It would be as well not to grin when the lady is by.

– o O o –

You must serve your time as agreed in the indentures, unless you can get another master to take you over for the rest of the apprenticeship.

– o O o –

AN ANXIOUS MOTHER – wishes to know 'if an ironmonger can compel his apprentices to be behind the counter till nine o'clock one evening, and ten another night.' In the absence of specified hours in the indentures, we should say that a master, whether ironmonger or not, would expect his apprentices' services during the usual hours of business. The hours mentioned certainly seem late, but there may be indulgences on the other side of which we know nothing. Speaking broadly, we should say that nothing will be gained by the apprentice standing too much upon his 'rights.' 'Better for a man that he wear the yoke in his youth.'

– o O o –

The provisions of the Factory Act vary with the age of the persons subject to it. A 'young person' – not necessarily an apprentice – is entitled to eight half-holidays between August and October, and to the whole of Christmas Day and Good Friday or another day in lieu of the latter.

– o O o –

TIRED OUT – It is simply cruel to work a boy seventy-six hours a week, but there is no law to put a stop to it. People who serve in shops have very long hours, and the smaller the shop the longer the hours for master as well as for men. The only way out of the difficulty is for you to get something else to do; and in changing you might go from bad to worse.

Many of the boys enquired about careers in the services, perhaps because the most popular serials in the paper were about adventures on the high seas, ocean-going trips round the world, or rugged exploits involving the firing of guns. But there were many hurdles to be overcome before a boy could put on the uniform he fancied. For one thing, he couldn't become a colonel straight away, and he might have to do a bit of fighting:

You must serve in the ranks. If you want to be a soldier, be a soldier, and if you are not prepared to take your share of the dangerous work stay away from the army altogether.

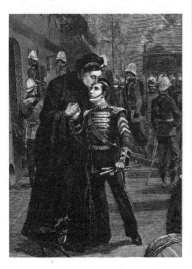

Surely you can see the absurdity of a man wanting all the distinction of the pretty uniform, all the certainty of the pay, and all the borrowed glory of the fighting men, of whom outsiders mistake him to be one – and at the same time doing merely penwork safely out of reach of annoyance or disturbance.

– oOo –

The Army does not want drummer boys that are afraid to go out of the country, so you had better give up the idea. Drummers are generally chosen by the colonels, or come from the bands in schools; they do *not* come from the Military School at Sandhurst.

– oOo –

R. M. 'wishes to know what height he must be to join the band of the 60th Rifles, and whether he must have a knowledge of music.' The bandsmen of most regiments are now obtained from the band companies of the various military and orphan schools – from lads who have not only been chosen from their fellows because of their special fitness, but who also have been trained as musicians from an early age. Outsiders would have little or no chance. Height is not a consideration in the bands. The height of the rank and file in the 60th Rifles is 5ft. 4 1/2 in.; and the chest measurement 34in.

– oOo –

You are not tall enough for the Cavalry. You might join the Artillery or the Transport Corps as a driver. Better wait a little longer – or rather grow a little longer. Get 'The Advantages of the Army' from the nearest post-office.

– oOo –

Judging from your writing and spelling, you would not have the remotest chance of passing at Sandhurst without some years of training. Would your age and means admit of this?

– oOo –

1. The chances of your receiving a commission are so remote that they are better disregarded. 2. Promotion in the infantry is no more rapid than in the cavalry. In neither service could you live comfortably on your pay. 3. All the so-called Highland regiments wear kilts. [*To show off their Highland legs?*]

– oOo –

You will never make a soldier. When a boy asks what time a soldier has to turn out in the morning, and what 'hours' he has to work, he is not even fit for the militia. Better give up all thoughts of 'The First Horse Life Guards.' The country could not afford to pay you 1s. 9d. a day, even if all of it were deducted 'in regards to living.'

– oOo –

The B.O.P. was particularly harsh on boys who wanted to join someone else's army:

To enlist in the Chilean army as a private soldier would be madness, even if they would accept you.

– o O o –

No, not unless you can speak the language, and even then your application would be looked upon with suspicion. If you want to be a soldier, join our army. Why join the French? Are you thinking of the field-marshal's baton that is said to form part of the contents of the conscript's knapsack?

– o O o –

We would not help you if we could. We have not an atom of sympathy for mercenaries, and consider English officers in Continental armies very much out of place. If you must fight, fight for Queen Victoria, and combine a little patriotism with your exuberant pugnacity.

– o O o –

We have no sympathy with English lads entering the combatant services of foreign powers. If you must fight, fight for your old country.

– o O o –

Many boys wanted to be sailors although, as the Editor told boys, there were certain physical requirements:

There is no medical examination for the merchant service; nevertheless, a very short-sighted person would be somewhat out of place at sea.

– o O o –

Apply to any of the institutes for the deaf and dumb. From their leading officials you would very probably get valuable hints and help. Your going to sea is quite out of the question. In all such cases of affliction it is well to apply to the establish-

ments that exist for their special treatment; they have patients of all incomes, and hence necessarily learn the various branches in which those that consult them can obtain employment.

– o O o –

BAD TOE – Yes; if it is much, and makes you in any way lame. How foolish to wear such tight boots! Be it known to you and all boys thinking of the Royal Navy that perfection of health and body are looked for. No knock-knees, no pigeon-breasts, no bad eyes, or bad teeth. The lad must be *crème de la crème.*

– o O o –

We could not say unless we saw you. Only the *crème de la crème* of boys are passed into the Royal Navy. We have known boys objected to because they were ugly in face and ungainly.

– o O o –

No; we don't think the decay of three teeth would disqualify for the Marines; but all would depend on the cause of the decay. Consult some medical officer.

– o O o –

PIGEON BREAST – No good for the Navy. Consult a surgeon.

– o O o –

The only rank – if it can be termed one – above paymaster is that of secretary to a commander-in-chief, flag-officer, or commodore. If you wish to go to sea, and do not care about making a fortune, by all means join that branch of the service. The highest pay – seldom reached – is about £590 per annum.

– o O o –

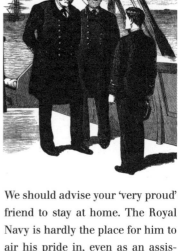

We should advise your 'very proud' friend to stay at home. The Royal Navy is hardly the place for him to air his pride in, even as an assistant-clerk. We do not know all that midshipmen look down upon nowadays, but they certainly would look down on such petty vanity as you describe.

– o O o –

Seventeen is rather too old for a boy to go for a sailor. 'At first go off' you would get nothing. You would be useless.

– o O o –

Get Mr. Stansfield Hicks on 'What to do with our Boys,' published by Wilson, of the Minories. It will give you full information as to the apprenticeship, pay, and prospects of marine engineers.

– o O o –

You will have to be apprenticed for about four years to an engineering firm where marine engines are made; then you ship as assistant-engineer; then you become certificated, and go as second engineer; and after a year's service you are eligible for a berth as chief engineer. You can go as engine-room boy on board ship, and get moved up to be fourth or third engineer, in which capacity you must serve four years before you are eligible to pass your first examination. But the first way is the best. Your apprenticeship should begin when you are about fifteen.

– o O o –

You are too old. 'A middy's bearth in the R. N.' will never come in your bill of fare. You will have to stay ashore and learn to spell.

– o O o –

You have confused two very different things. A midshipman, or rather a cadet, has two chests, one in which he puts his clothes, the other which is measured by the

doctors, and which is used for quite other purposes.

– o O o –

If you want to go to sea, pray go; but let it be with the consent of your guardians. It is a hard life; but all life is hard, and there is not a trade or profession on land which is not one long struggle. The food of a sailor is both in practice and by law better than that of the class from which he comes. But at the same time remember you will be as much a 'slave' and 'prisoner' in a ship as you are in a workshop; it is all a question of opinion and descriptive terms.

– o O o –

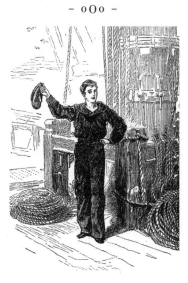

A 'Constant Reader' who writes to know how to join the Britannia at the very time a series of articles on that subject by a Lord of the Admiralty is running in the paper, must be too unintelligent to stand a chance in any examination whatsoever.

Part of the attraction of the armed services was the possibility of travel. Other boys sought to see the world in another way, by capitalising on the fact that Britain still had a large Empire, which needed civil servants and white immigrants to run the countries it had conquered or colonised:

Assisted passages are given to respectable men and women on the understanding that they come to the colony for good, and have no intention of returning. If your idea is to go to one of the colonies for a year or two and then come back, you had far better stay at home. You are not the sort of immigrant that the colonials would appreciate, and your availing yourself of their help simply to inspect them would be, in plain English, a fraud. You will live a far nobler and better life in this world if you regulate your conduct more by the spirit of justice and less by the letter of the law.

– oOo –

Your brother would seem to belong to the 'six of one and half dozen of the other' school, who never did anything in this world, and never will. There is no reason at all why you should not accept your uncle's invitation, pay your passage out, and look for work if necessary when you have visited your friends. You would have at least as much chance of work in the colonies as here. It is but a poor spirit that declines a friend's help when the help is honestly tendered. Take advantage of the offer, do not abuse it, and in the future help others as you have been helped.

– oOo –

The wonderful prophecy of the future greatness of Australia – 'Where Sydney Cove,' etc. – was written in 1790 by Dr. Erasmus Darwin.

– oOo –

The only way we can suggest for you to increase your growth to army height is to emigrate to Australia. It often happens that lads who have apparently stopped growing in this country take a fresh start under the sun of the Antipodes.

– oOo –

Go by all means, and when you get there never write to an editor and 'expect a satisfactory reply.' The Canadian Offices are at 9, Victoria Chambers, S.W.

– oOo –

A strange training for emigration – can stand rough treatment, 'as we have been used to it at home, on account of having a very unkind father.' – Poor boys! But go to one of our own colonies, to Tasmania, or another of the Australasian group, to which the passage is long enough for you to be of use. You might get out as steward's boys, at a nominal wage of a shilling a month, perhaps, as has been done lately by one or two lads of our acquaintance. But you will have to do dirty work morning, noon and night. We are officially informed that there is no opening for anyone on the Government Railways of Cape Colony, or in any of the Government services.

– oOo –

You would do better in Canada as a farmer than you would here as a clerk; but if you go to Canada it would be wise for you to work at wages for three or four years, and say nothing about the money you possess. When you have experience you can invest your money to advantage.

For boys who were happy to stay on dry land and in their own country, there was a range of careers. But the B.O.P. couldn't be encouraging about one very popular option:

CIVIL SERVICE – The social position is not worth mentioning, and the life is one of genteel poverty. You would be much better off as an artisan. There is no chance of an improvement in the prospects of the Civil Service so long as such crowds flock to the examinations, attracted by the commencing salary.

– oOo –

We decline to answer party questions. At the same time we think a little more thought would lead you to see the absurdity of inveighing on one page against Government 'extravagance,' and on the other proclaiming your intention of entering the Civil Service, 'where the salaries are so good and there is a pension'!!! Surely in a question, as you put it, of 'robbing taxpayers,' the receiver would be as bad as the thief.

– oOo –

Surely you must see that any well-regulated State can only employ as public servants those who are sound in sense and limb. If you were to look at these matters from a taxpayer's point of view instead of that of a Civil Service candidate, you would appreciate the reason why the maimed, the deaf, the halt, and the blind stand little chance of earning the nation's money. Your country wants for her servants her best men. It may suit your selfish purpose to 'dodge the doctor,' but please to remember that you thereby commit a fraud on those who are taxed to pay you your wages.

For the most part, the B.O.P. had to tell boys that the image they had of a particular career path was often wide of the mark:

Our candid opinion is that a near-sighted total-abstaining exciseman would not achieve any remarkable measure of success, and that he had far better turn his attention to something else.

– oOo –

You would stand little or no chance, we fear, of becoming a war correspondent for any of the dailies without first having made your mark as a writer on the staff, and given tangible proof of special aptitude for the work. Some experience of foreign travel, and an intimate knowledge of at least French and German, would be almost indispensable.

– oOo –

Your writing would be considered fairly good for commercial purposes; it is not firm and bold enough for the law.

– oOo –

Your 'riting' would probably answer for ordinary office work, but your spelling 'ergently' requires improvement.

– oOo –

Yes, you will have to become 'an ordinary policeman' first – a very ordinary policeman, we should say, judging from your handwriting.

– o O o –

Get a Whitakers Almanac, and see the name of the governor of the prison in which you wish to obtain an appointment. We do not think, however, you have the slightest chance of success.

– o O o –

Prison warders are generally old soldiers. Application should be made to the governor of the prison. No governor would do you the injustice to employ you.

– o O o –

'How to get on the stage?' We should very strongly and seriously recommend you to keep off it.

– o O o –

We strongly advise you to choose another trade. In an actor's calling, taking it at its best, and saying nothing of its associations, there are so many blanks to the few prizes that it is more of a starving than a living to thousands that follow it. You may of course have the exceptional ability that may bring you to the front, but, judging from your letter, we should think that the very reverse was the case.

– o O o –

Unless you have a gift for teaching, give up all thoughts of becoming a school-master. To say nothing of your life being a misery to yourself, think of the sufferings of your pupils!

And for a blessed few readers, their future was secured by a healthy bank balance. But even that presented problems which the Editor was asked to help with:

The only way is to buy Bank Stock, of which you will sometimes see the quotation in the Money Market column. By far the best plan, when you have too much for the Post Office Savings Bank, is to invest in Consols, which you can do for small amounts more easily through the Post Office than in any other way. A paper of instructions will be given you free on application at any post-office.

Chapter 6

=X=

'WE HAVE SO MANY LOVERS'

Portrait of 'the Editor'

I HAVE written of 'the Editor' as if it was one person who wrote the replies to all the correspondents. In fact, we know that the task was shared, probably on the basis of special interests – Dr. Stables on health and pets, the Rev. J.G. Wood on natural history, G.A. Hutchison, the actual editor, on B.O.P. matters, and W.J. Gordon – known to his colleagues as 'Fleet Street's walking encyclopaedia' – on almost everything else. But a kind of composite figure emerges from the odd personal glimpses slipped into answers, as well as the tone of intelligence, wit and playfulness that – on a good day – the answers contain.

Let's start with the various personal details the Editor let slip in his answers. He usually used the royal 'we':

To stop screw-holes in your boot-heel use cobbler's-wax. We have always found our screw-holes to stop up much too quickly of themselves, and the difficulty has been to clear them out.

– oOo –

We are very much obliged for your offer of a live sea-gull from your district, and have no doubt it will arrive safely. We shall certainly keep it in memory of the sender.

We should not object to receive one from other places round our British and Irish coasts, or even from the colonies. We greatly treasure the horns, leaves, plants, etc., we have received from distant readers. A small 'Christmas Bush' (*Ceratopetalum gummiferum*) sent us from Sydney unfortunately arrived quite dead, having been damaged with salt water.

– oOo –

You have probably gone on the usual, but wrong, principle in your Turkish baths. Instead of beginning at a moderate temperature, and increasing it gradually, do just the reverse. Do not eat anything for at least two hours before you bathe. Walk at your best pace to the bath, go at once into the highest temperature which you can endure, stay there as long as you can, and then move into the cooler rooms. This plan was taught us by Mr. Urquhart himself. We have taken six Turkish baths in a week, and found the greatest benefit from them. As for temperature, we prefer 240 degrees or thereabouts for the first room, and 140 for the last but one. Until we took Mr. Urquhart's advice, we always had a headache on leaving the bath, but after following it, we have often entered with a headache, and left without it. Still, this plan may not suit every one, as constitutions differ.

– o O o –

The Lubeck Infant was Christian Henry Heinecken, who at one year old knew the chief events of the Mosaic books, at thirteen months knew all Old Testament history, in another month knew all about the New Testament, at two years and a half could answer any ordinary question in history or geography, at three years old knew well both French and Latin, and at four years old died – just before he was sufficiently accomplished to answer the correspondence of the BOY'S OWN PAPER!

– o O o –

Correspondents are not expected to forward locks of their hair, even when of such a lovely golden brown as yours.

– o O o –

J. R. F. asks. 'Which is the best time to bathe? Early in the morning, at noon, or in the evening?'... If you are in good health you may bathe at any time, except just after a meal or when very fatigued. We have a friend, and not a particularly young one either, who often enjoys a midnight swim by moonlight.

– o O o –

You could get a second-hand cornet at one of Puttnick and Simpson's auction sales, or at any of the second-hand general shops, of which there are so many about. A second-hand wind instrument does not seem a pleasant invest-ment, though we suppose it is only a fancy of ours. Don't you think you had better get a new mouth-piece?

– oOo –

A correspondent, whose letter we have unfortunately mislaid, sent us some little time ago a large green caterpillar, which he had found in a potato-field ...

– oOo –

You should write to some maga-zine which treats cricket with contempt. The difficulty never occurred to us. All the wives, and the sisters, and the cousins, and the aunts of every one connected with the BOY'S OWN PAPER take a considerable amount of interest in cricket, and never behave them-selves in *that* way!

– oOo –

Publish your letter? Not for the world! Though it is the biggest we ever had – we thought you had sent us a table-cloth by mistake.

– oOo –

Impossible to say. Our idea of a man is one six feet high, with

shoulders to match, but many people would be satisfied with smaller specimens. Stature and growth vary so much under climate and conditions.

– oOo –

We could ride on a bicycle from Stamford Hill to Walton-on-the-Naze in a day, but we have no means of knowing if you could. The best map is the Ordnance Survey Map, an inch to the mile. The other maps are made up from it, and you might just as well have the original.

– oOo –

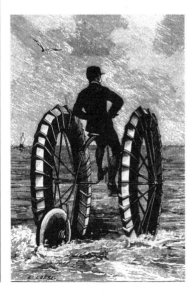

Boys are often apt both to talk and walk in their sleep, but they quickly lose these habits as they grow up. A few months ago we were startled in the dead of night by a young lad who had, while asleep, made his way into our room, and, after trying on our boots, wanted to get into our bed. He will probably lose the habit of sleep-walking after his fright on awakening.

– oOo –

LOVER OF B.O.P. – Choose a different *nom de plume* next. We have so many lovers.

The next few answers show 'the Editor's' personal interest in natural history.

We do not think you will be successful in entrapping the shrew-mouse. You say you hear them. When we were as young as you we did not content ourselves with hearing them. We boldly pulled the grass about, and often made a capture. By all means let us hear how you get on in the 'mice fancy.'

– oOo –

We had a pet chameleon in Africa once; he dined on insects, and sometimes he did not dine for a week on a stretch. He had the gout, perhaps. He lived in a coffee pot, and the cockroaches and he did not seem to pull well together. Give your pet sunshine, anyhow, and the means of retirement.

– oOo –

Your glowworms were probably eaten by toads; we once lost nearly fifty in a couple of nights in just the same way. They feed, as grubs, upon snails, of which each is said to devour three, and therefore in some small degree they are useful to mankind. You will find a full description, etc., in 'Our Insect Allies,' by Mr. Theodore Wood, published at 2s. 6d.

– oOo –

Hedgehogs should be provided with their ordinary food, which is always of an animal nature. Their semi-hibernating habits cause some trouble in keeping them. We have possessed several, and although, in consequence of the perpetual supply of cockroaches, they postponed hibernation as long as possible, they always contrived to get out of the house before the winter was over, and hid themselves in a large tool-shed, which was filled with pea-sticks and bean-sticks almost to the roof.

– o O o –

The name of your female dog must be left to your own discretion: we know one which actually answers to 'Tommy'!

– o O o –

You are Bland, so are we, else we would not write you a short article on the Aquarium; but it is Christmas time, so for once in a way we obey.... [*A 225-word account follows, and the answer ends:*] We cannot spare more space; but the getting-up of an aquarium is a most delightful fancy, and well repays the trouble. Read the capital articles on the subject by the Rev. J.G. Wood, that

have already appeared in our columns.

– o O o –

We cannot at present spare Dr. Gordon Stables to go so far as Jamaica to see your poor Polly, though he himself would, he says, 'go like a shot.' Give the bird nothing but seeds, grain, and nuts, with now and then a chilli. Rub the sore places with Vaseline; give a bath. Yes, a fowl put in solitary confinement for a time in the dark will go off the 'cluck.'

– o O o –

Had you read our pigeon articles you would not now have written. But do not imagine that we think it any trouble to answer our boys. It is a pleasure.

– o O o –

Buried in a few of the answers, consistently over the first decade or so, at least, is a sly delight in wordplay, wit and, occasionally, sarcasm. This can be a dangerous technique. Used to reading serious and informative replies on pets, hobbies and general knowledge, how is a boy to know his leg is being pulled, as it sometimes was, or even to recognise the kind of joke that pater would never make? When a boy wrote in about his blackheads and called them 'flesh worms' the reply was:

The 'flesh worms' in your nose are a remarkable variety of spider! With the point of a needle work round the little dark spot. You can then squeeze them out by the two thumb-nails.

Would every boy reading that reply know that it was a joke? But other replies were more obvious, and sometimes quite witty.

1. We do not know 'how to make a photographer transperant for the magic-lantern;' though our house-maid declares she soon 'saw through' one who wanted to get into our front garden and take her *carte*.

– o O o –

What is the use of our giving articles on electric lamps if we are to receive such queries as yours while these articles are appearing? You might at least buy the *current* numbers.

– o O o –

We should think a watchmaker would find it difficult to get a living in Patagonia; but perhaps the fact of no other watchmaker having thought of going there might be in his favour. You would find it a far safer escapement to Australia.

– o O o –

How to add a human skull to your collection? Perhaps the hospital authorities could advise you, or perhaps you could get one from the natural history shops. Why not use your own for the purpose?

– o O o –

Your query reminds us of the examination story of the candidate who was asked what was the cost of a ton of tea at ninepence per pound, and who was plucked because, instead of working out the question, he sagely replied, 'You can't get tea at the price, and I don't see the use of wasting time about such rubbish!'

– o O o –

A CONSTANT READER simply says: 'Dear Sir, – Will you kindly grant me the favour of explaining in correspondence in the BOY'S OWN PAPER the origin of our surname?' It would be a melancholy satisfaction for us to do so if we could. It is said that an American lady could never imagine where all the Smiths came from until in a town in Massachusetts she came across 'The Smith Manufacturing Company:' and we rather incline to the opinion that in some secluded spot there must be 'A Constant Reader Manufacturing Company,' unlim-ited, who turn out so many circu-lars per week, of which we, as in duty bound, receive our full share!

– o O o –

Conscience-money is money sent to the Chancellor of the Exchequer by conscience-stricken individuals who have found it impossible to support any longer the whole of the weight of guilt at having misled the income-tax assessors, and so relieve themselves by sending in a trifle on account.

– o O o –

Chimney-pot hats are not usually worn at sea. You might find one useful, however, in case of shipwreck, if you were to tie a handkerchief over it and use it, brim downwards, as a life-buoy. We do not know 'why looking-glasses are put into cheap hats,' unless it be to show the wearers how badly they fit! The 'holes round them' may be for 'sweetness and light'!

– o O o –

Surely you can see that it is an error of the press, wherein 'miles' has been substituted for 'yards.' Write to the publishers or printers. You will probably receive a similar reply to that given by the Cleveland editor who, when it was pointed out that his paper said a hill in Japan was 500 miles high, came out in his next issue with, 'We regret that, by an error of the press, the height of the hill in Japan was exaggerated. Readers are requested to deduct 2,639,500 feet from the former statement.'

– o O o –

We are not sure of the colour of the South-Eastern Railway carriages. The paint is rarely visible owing to the thick covering of dirt by which it is concealed. The best plan would be to get a porter to wash a panel or so for you. We have some recollection of once seeing a new carriage painted plum-colour – but would rather not commit ourselves.

– o O o –

Lothbury is the street alongside the Bank of England; but we cannot tell you the age of the clock. The particulars you give remind us of the problem in navigation – Given the price of the captain's shoe-buckles: required – the latitude of the ship.

– o O o –

We do not treat such questions 'seriously,' because we have no means of knowing if they are asked in good faith. Is it likely that any person with the slightest pretentions to sense would ask a stranger how 'to soften the bone of his nose' so that he can 'mould it into a better shape'? Here is one personage wishing to know how to 'force' a moustache; and from Cardiff we have a specimen letter asking if the nose can be improved by rubbing it, if whiskers will drop out at twenty when left alone, and if there is an oil 'to anoint the hair with' which will put the break on so that the querist need never visit the barber. 'T.K.' wishes to know how he is to raise his hat to a lady when he has both hands full. Another hero, 'Agamemnon' his name, wishes to know, 'Can a person reduce superfluous flesh by drinking vinegar?' Perhaps he would like to increase his by no means superfluous brain by eating the same liquid with a fork!

– oOo –

Certainly. The 'best plan for extracting Indian ink from the body through the B.O.P.' is to unfold the paper and lay it on the skin with this answer against the part affected! Then get a companion to press slowly and with deliberation over the part with a hot flat-iron until the Indian ink fades away to the extent required!

– oOo –

For instructions in the management of calves consult some dairy manual, or apply to some agricultural newspaper. Since writing this it has occurred to us that perhaps you mean the calves on your legs. If so, we are unable to tell you how to 'grow them'. We believe that their abnormal development is a trade secret, never communicated previous to the assumption of the plush!

– oOo –

We are not responsible for the opinions of 'other papers.' If you doubt that you weigh more after a meal than before it, a very simple experiment will enlighten you. Your argument simply leads you to the conclusion that the more you eat the less you weigh, and you have only to keep on eating to weigh nothing. As to 'the air displaced by the food weighing more than the food which has taken its place,' apart from the difficulty of getting our food down, we should if it were true have our legs of mutton flying upwards like balloons, and be obliged to keep our joints and puddings guyed to the tablecloth to prevent their shooting off into space.

– oOo –

'A short time ago, thinking that my moustache did not grow satisfactorily, I shaved it off, fancying it would in consequence be stronger. I now find that the right side grows faster than the other.' This is a new version of the 'Hair and the Tortoise.' Patience, O Distressed One! The race is not always to the swift.

– oOo –

We would rather not give an article on 'How to Shave Yourself.' Our intentions might be misunderstood, as we should have to illustrate with cuts, and that would raise a laugh at the shaver's expense! [*Cuts = woodcuts, and by extension any engraved illustration.*]

– oOo –

Do not interfere with moles, whether they appear on the skin or work in the garden or field.

– oOo –

Did you ever read the 'Emperor's New Clothes,' a Scandinavian story? If not, do so. Sampson Low and Co. publish it at sixpence. Making 'invisible ink' will be very much the same sort of thing as described in that little book. We have given instructions many times about inks that will appear and disappear, if that is what you want. There was a patent taken out in America some time ago for an ink that faded entirely, and a lawsuit ensued thereupon. A merchant had bought the secret from the patentee, and paid for it in bills at six months. The inventor kept the bills, and when he went to present them, lo! they were but pieces of blank paper. *They had been written in his own ink!*

– oOo –

INVISIBLE INK RECIPE – We regret the delay. It may be, however, that the printer printed the answer in the ink you require, and that it has passed us unknown. Pray hold out the last year's numbers to the fire, and see if you can warm up the desired reply.

– oOo –

UMSLOPOGAAS says that he has often held a kettle of boiling water on his hand, 'but it is absolutely necessary that the bottom should be covered with soot; carbon being a very bad conductor of heat, does not allow the warmth of boiling water to come to the hand.' And he thinks this is worthy of a place in *Quicquid agunt pueri nostri farrago libelli*, which means that 'The book is about whatever is of interest to boys,' and was provided by Juvenal. Now, Umslop., cease to be haggard! [*Umslopogaas was a character in two novels by H. Rider Haggard.*]

– o O o –

1. What an examiner you would make! 'The teacher says that anything with life in it is masculine or feminine gender. I want to know, if you were parsing the sentence, 'Mr. Wilson is dead,' would Mr. Wilson be neuter gender?' Clearly the teacher should have given the other side of the question, and you would have parsed Mr. Wilson as masculine without misgiving. 2. 'Is all ancient history true?' Well, as we can personally vouch for all modern history not being true, we must decline to guarantee the accuracy of the somewhat contradictory statements of the ancients. 3.

Perhaps the cornet, but authorities differ.

– o O o –

1. It is currently reported that a cuckoo lays its own eggs, but we cannot personally vouch for the fact. We are content to take the statement on trust. 2. Why not try the experiment? It is not usual to hard-boil a bird's egg before you blow it, but we live and learn, and you might solve what to others may seem an impossibility. If you *do* succeed in blowing a hard-boiled egg we shall be glad to hear full particulars as to how you managed it!

– o O o –

Your meaning is not very clear. If you mean *you* have got a tail, you can curl it whichever way you please. If it is your dog who has the curly tail, he has similar freedom of choice in the matter.

– o O o –

As the dog seems so extremely susceptible you had better remove him. If there is much whitewash about he might catch the distemper(!).

– o O o –

...the question emanated from Colney Hatch. If you multiply a gallon of pitch by a quart of peri-winkles, what is the result? [*Colney Hatch was a North London lunatic asylum.*]

– oOo –

We must frankly confess our inability to suggest satisfactory treatment for a hare that has gone out of its mind, and 'jumps over everything that it comes to, however high.' Does it jump over churches? Does it clear steeples? It ought to be invaluable as a steeple-chaser. Mark Twain's jumping frog cannot be a circumstance to it. Do not send it to our office, please, it might be inconvenient, but write to the medical superintendent at Hanwell. He might take it there. [*Hanwell was another asylum near London.*]

– oOo –

Seems to us you are step-uncle to the baby. We cannot get any nearer than that. Our considering cap has gone to be repaired. We will try to give hints now and then in our Queer Pets paragraph about Aquarium. A paper on the Vivarium is being prepared by Dr. Gordon Stables.

– oOo –

Dear William, we are not a wizard. How can we tell why your Nanny scratches if you do not give us all particulars. You are only one of many who write us thus. Perhaps she is badly bedded. Perhaps she is thinking. Perhaps she is going to write a story for the B.O.P.!

– oOo –

Thanks, many thanks, but you are hopelessly wrong all the same:-

> Teach not a parent's parent to extract
> The golden juices of the egg by suction;
> The good old lady can the feat enact
> Quite irrespective of your kind instruction!

– oOo –

We really could not take on ourselves the responsibility of explaining to you 'how to destroy aunts,' however downtrodden a nephew you may be. If you mean 'ants,' dip pieces of sponge into diluted treacle, and place them into your cupboards till the insects have crowded into them, when you can drop them into boiling water.

– oOo –

No one has yet succeeded in 'bringing out a perpetual motion,' nor is it likely any prize would be offered for what no one would live long enough to prove.

– oOo –

The steeple is the whole thing, tower and all; the spire begins at the top of the tower. Many Nonconformist places of worship have steeples, and the saying you quote is a popular delusion. The old story of the tall boy whose mother intended him for the Church, and whose aunt thought she intended him for the steeple, might have put you on the right track.

– oOo –

Why, certainly! Thanks for the riddles; no 'exuze' necessary. They are not indigenous to African soil, but have probably been imported to make the proverbial Kaffir laugh. However, here they are – 'I went to India, but I did not go there; I came back because I stopped there. The answer is, 'a watch,' you understand?' The next is – 'Everything has what a German sausage has, or a German sausage has what everything else has. The answer is, 'a name.' Out here there was £5 offered for the right answer to that, and nobody guessed it. There's another one, but–' Well, it has not got quite the right tone about it better not. Send us some more, Bailey, but let them be of native growth. Give us an example from the place near you, where there are no eggs, owing to the natives having extirpated the whites, and thrown off their yolk!

– oOo –

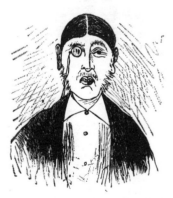

An Upper Story to let – unfurnished!

SCIENCE AND TECHNOLOGY

FACTS ABOUT GEMS

There are two gem alphabets in common use – one of transparent stones, the other of opaque ones. The transparent stones are – amethyst, beryl, chrysoberyl, diamond, emerald, fluorspar, garnet, hyacinth, idocrase, kyanite, lynx-sapphire, milk-opal, natrolite, opal, pyrope, quartz, ruby, sapphire, topaz, uranite, vesuvianite, water-sapphire, xanthite, zircon. The opaque series is – agate, basalt, cacholong, diaspore, Egyptian pebble, fire-blende, girasol, heliotrope, jasper, krokidolite, lapis lazuli, malachite, nephrite, onyx, porphyry, quartz-agate, rose-quartz, sardonyx, turquoise, ultramarine, verd-antique, wood opal, xylotile, zurlite. Substitutes for many of these you can easily find.

The apostolic jewels are – Andrew, a sapphire; Bartholomew, a red carnelian; James the Great, a white chalcedony; James the Less, a topaz; John, an emerald; Matthew, an amethyst; Matthias, a chrysolite; Peter, a jasper; Philip, a sardonyx; Simeon, a pink hyacinth; Thaddeus, a chrysoprase; Thomas, a beryl – as emblematic respectively of faith, martyrdom, purity, delicacy, gentleness, sobriety, truth, solidity, amiability, kindness, serenity, and cautiousness.

SOLAR SYSTEM IN FRUIT AND VEG

To include the whole solar system you would require a space like Hyde Park and Kensington Gardens together. At Hyde Park Corner you would have the sun represented by a globe two feet in diameter. At a distance of eighty-two feet you would have Mercury represented by a grain of mustard-seed. Sixty feet further from that you would have Venus represented by a pea. At a distance of 215 feet from the sun you would have the earth, also represented by a pea. At 327 feet from the sun you would have Mars as big as a peppercorn. Then, for the minor planets, you could dust down five or six hundred grains of sand. A quarter of a mile from the sun Jupiter would be represented by an orange. Two-fifths of a mile from the sun would come Saturn, represented by a small orange. Three-quarters of a mile from Hyde Park Corner, Uranus would be the size of a cherry; and half a mile further away you would have Neptune, as big as a plum. Having arranged your field, you could make the objects show the daily motion by moving them at the following rates each day: Mercury 3 feet a day, Venus 2 feet, the earth $1^7/_8$ feet, Mars $1^1/_2$ feet, Jupiter $10^1/_2$ inches, Saturn $7^1/_2$ inches, Uranus 5 inches, and Neptune 4 inches. The remembrance of Neptune as big as a plum revolving at the distance of a mile and a quarter from a two-feet sun at the rate of four inches a day, will give you as good a notion as you are likely to get of the magnitude of the solar system.

BABBAGE'S CALCULATING ENGINE

Babbage's first model was completed in 1822. The Government heard of it through the Royal Society, and made periodical advances towards the construction of a machine. In 1834 only a portion was ready, and as the Government had already advanced £17,000 (over and above what the inventor had himself spent on it, besides giving his own superintendence without remuneration), and saw no definite limit to the amount it would cost, the supplies were discontinued, and the machine remained unfinished. Had the engine been completed it would have had columns for six orders of differences, each of twenty places of figures, whilst the first three columns would have had half a dozen additional figures.

SUN FALLACY

We do not know why the sun puts a fire out; because, as a matter of fact, the sun does not put out a fire. It is probably a delusion. The placing of a poker on the top of the fire to draw it up is another popular absurdity, and is the relic of the old superstition which led people to make a cross over the fire so as to scare away the evil spirits which were supposed to be in it. Your questions are of the same character as the one addressed by the King Charles II to the Royal Society, when he asked for the reason why a bucketful of water with live fish in it weighed no more than the same quantity of water without the fish.

SHOT STORY

Shot is made by pouring melted lead through a colander into a cistern many feet below. Hence the necessity of shot towers like those near Waterloo Bridge. The making of shot in this way was invented in 1782 by a plumber of Bristol named Watts, who went to sleep and dreamt he was out in a shower of rain in which the clouds sent down lead instead of water, and the lead was in small spheres. Thinking he might make shot in this way, he ascended to the top of St. Mary Redcliffe Church with his ladle, and then, melting some lead, he poured it into the water he had placed on the pavement.

NATURE

EVER HOPFUL

Cuckoo-spit is formed by a homopterous insect known as *Aprophora Spumaria*, belonging to the *Cecropidae* or Hopper family. Its popular name is the Froghopper, from the fact of its jumping enormous distances in proportion to its size, making the leaves click as it takes off, and frequently landing sprawling on its back and righting itself after a pause – much on the principle of Sir Wilfrid Lawson's Yankee, who arrived on the pier as the steamer was moving off, and just caught his toe in the taffrail and landed on his head on the steamer's deck, where he came to after a quarter of an hour or so, during which the land had been left some distance behind, and, raising himself on his hands, looked across the intervening space and exclaimed in astonishment, 'Jehoshaphat! what a jump!' The larva feeds on various plants, and sucks their juices through the long tubular beak which in some species in this family is nearly as long as the body. In the heat of the day, and when the accumulation is greatest, a drop of clear water begins to form at the lowest part of the deposit, and the froth drains into it, and falls eventually to the ground. There is a Madagascar species, *Aprophora Goudotii*, which pours out clear water and has no froth.

DROP THE DEAD DONKEY

It is all nonsense about dead donkeys being never seen. They are not left where they die, any more than horses or men are. As to the age attainable by donkeys (four-footed ones) we are not able to reply; we mean as to the extreme limit. In an article on 'The Age of Animals' in January part, 1870, of the 'Leisure Hour,' it is stated that the horse and the ass, in domestic state do not often live longer than from twenty to twenty-five years. Old age prostrated 'Copenhagen,' the Duke of Wellington's famous charger, at twenty-seven years. There are cases on record of far greater age, and probably the age of the ass is also sometimes prolonged.

TALL OLD TREES

The highest trees in the world, as far as at present known, grow in California, at Big Tree Creek and other places. They are

Sequoia giganteas, and run from 275ft. to 376ft. high, and from 25ft. to 34ft. in diameter. One there was carefully measured at 106ft. in circumference at its base, and 76ft. at 12ft. from the ground. They are from two to three thousand years old. The oldest trees in the world are said to be the Baobab of Senegal, the Dragon-tree of Orotava, the Cypress of Chapultepec, the Chestnuts of Etna, and the Plane at Bujukdere, near Constantinople, all estimated at over 5,000 years. Darnoy's Oak in Dorsetshire is 2,000 years of age, the Winfarthing Oak in Norfolk, and the Bentley Oak, were more than 700 years old at the Conquest. Cowthorpe Oak, near Wetherby, is 1,600 years old. The Bull Oak at Wedgenock Park, and the Plester Oak at Colborne, existed long previous to Edward the Confessor. Wallace's Oak at Paisley is 700 years old. Owen Glendower's Oak at Shelton is the very tree from whose branches he watched the battle of Shrewsbury in 1403. Braburn Yew is 3,000 years old. Fortingal Yew, in Perthshire, about the same. Darley Yew, in Derbyshire, over 2,000 years. Crowhurst Yew, in Surrey, at least 1,400 years; and the three yews at Fountains Abbey are the trees under which the abbey founders arranged its plans at a solemn picnic they held there in 1132.

CHICKEN FACTS

The old scale of points for judging Spangled Hamburg hens is as follows (want of space prevents us treating your queries more fully). The scale does for both silver and golden varieties, by altering the ground colour. Comb – best double, best square, most erect, and piked behind. Ears – largest and most white. Neck – best streaked with greenish black in middle of feathers, and best fringed with gold at edges. Breast, back, and rump – largest moons, best and brightest greenish black, most free from white tips at end of moons, and clearest and best red from moons to bottom colour. Wing – its bow, best and brightest greenish black and clearest red; its bars two in number, distinct, and of largest, clearest, brightest, and best greenish black; moons best greenish black, and of clearest and best red; its stepping with largest, clearest, brightest, and best greenish black spots on ends of feathers, and with best and clearest red from spots to bottom colour. Tail – fullest feathered, brightest, darkest, and best greenish black. Legs – best and clearest blue. General appearance – the best-feathered hen.

SHOCKING STORY

Perhaps you mean *Elsassia electrica*, the electrical tree. The report goes that during their recent exploration of north-east New Guinea, Lieutenant Himmergosende and Dr. Kummel reached a spot twelve days' journey from the coast where their compass became useless owing to the presence of a tree which possessed the properties of a highly charged electrical battery, and that Dr. Kummel was knocked down when he touched the trunk. Somehow it was chopped at, however, and on analysis proved to be almost pure amorphous carbon. We do not vouch for the truth of this shocking story, which is said to have originated in the 'South Australian Advertiser.'

NOISES OFF

A cuckoo cries, we suppose. There is no need to coin a verb to cuckoo. A magpie chatters. You may as well have a list and choose for yourself. Here is a fairly full one: – Apes gibber, asses bray, bees hum, beetles drone, bears growl, bitterns boom, blackbirds whistle, bullfinches pipe, bulls bellow, canaries sing, cats mew and purr, calves bleat, chaffinches chirp, chickens peep, cocks crow, cows low or moo, crows caw, dogs bark, bay, howl, or yelp; doves coo, ducks quack, eagles scream, falcons chant, flies buzz, foxes bark and yelp, frogs croak, geese cackle, grasshoppers chirp, grouse drum, guinea-pigs squeak, gulls scream, hawks scream, hens cluck, horses neigh and whinney, hyaenas laugh, jays chatter, lambs bleat, larks sing, linnets chuckle, lions roar, mice squeal, monkeys chatter, nightingales pipe and warble, owls hoot and screech, parrots talk, peacocks scream, pigeons coo, pigs grunt, squeak, and squeal; plovers cry peewit, ravens croak, redstarts whistle, rooks caw, sheep baa or bleat, snakes hiss, sparrows chirrup, swallows twitter, swans cry, thrushes whistle, tigers growl, turkeys gobble, vultures scream, whitethroats chirr, wolves howl, and yellowhammers call 'a little bit of bread and no cheese.'

THIS MODERN WORLD

ENGINE LIGHTS

The lights on an engine are to show the railway men to what stations the train is bound. The position varies with the different destinations of the trains, and the discs by day take the place of the lamps by night. On the District Railway, for instance, a single lamp to the left proclaims the mainline train to Aldgate, a lamp at each side distinguishes a Hammersmith train, two lamps one over the other in the middle show an Addison Road train, three lamps all of a horizontal row a Putney train, three lamps arranged triangularly an Ealing train, two lamps diagonally a Willesden train, and three lamps – two to the left one over the other and one to the right – proclaim the train to Richmond.

RAILWAY FACTS

It was the Midland Railway Company that first resolved to run only first and third class to all trains, and there has been no second class on the line for years. The suggestion is said to have come from Sir James Allport, who was then general manager of the company.

It is not true that the life of a railway servant is more dangerous than it used to be. In the four years ending 1869 the Mutual Assurance Society on the Great Western show four deaths and three disablements per thousand; while in the four years ending 1884 the deaths have sunk to 1.3 and the disablements to 1.1 per thousand.

The North-Western foot-warmers are filled with acetate of soda instead of water. The acetate melts at about the boiling point of water, and it is melted in the sealed case before being used. As it cools it crystallises, and throws out the latent heat.

Accidents occur everywhere, but the number of deaths from accident are comparatively few when compared with the total deaths from all causes. It has been calculated from official and elaborate data by one of the most eminent of living statisticians, that if a person were to live continually in a railway carriage, and spend all his time in railway travelling, the chance in favour of his dying from a railway accident would not occur until he had been rushing along the lines for nine hundred and sixty years! The average express speed in England is said to be fifty miles an hour, in Belgium forty-one, in France and Germany thirty-nine, in Italy thirty-one, and in Austria, Russia, and Switzerland twenty-seven.

BUSBY-BAGS

The following are the colours of the busby-bags of our Hussar regiments: Blue for the 3rd and the 18th; yellow for the 4th and 14th; scarlet for the 7th and 8th; red for the 10th and 15th; crimson for the 11th and 20th; buff for the 13th; white for the 19th; and grey for the 21st. The plume of the 3rd is white, that of the

18th is red and white; the plume of the 4th is scarlet, that of the 14th is white; the plume of the 7th is white, that of the 8th is red and white; the plume of the 10th is black and white, that of the 15th is red; and the plume of the 11th is crimson and white, while that of the 20th is crimson.

LARGE AD

The largest single advertisement in the world is said to be the annual printing of the list of delinquent taxpayers in Cook County, Illinois. According to a special enactment, those who fail to pay their taxes in that county have to have 'their names in alphabetical order published in the public press,' and this is met by inserting them once as an advertisement in the 'Chicago Tribune.' The list extends to six hundred and sixteen columns, and costs over three thousand pounds!

TEA MATTERS

TEETOTALER – Nothing whatever to do with tea. The term is due to the fact that in the early days of the temperance movement one of the orators at a large meeting in Lancashire unfortunately stuttered somewhat, and in speaking of total abstinence pronounced it 't-t-t-total abstinence.' Hence in derision his supporters were nicknamed 't-t-t-totalers' or 'teetotalers,' and that nickname has now lost its sting and become classical English.

RULE OF THE ROAD

The rule of the road in this country is the exact opposite to what it is on the Continent. There you keep to the right hand; here:

> The rule of the road is a paradox quite,
> If you keep to the left you are sure to be right.

ARMS AND THE MEN

There are three English Kings-at-Arms: Garter, Clarencieux, and Norroy; six Heralds: Chester, Lancaster, York, Somerset, Richmond, and Windsor, besides a 'Surrey Extraordinary' and a 'Maltravers Extra,' whatever they may be. There are also four Pursuivants: Rouge Croix, Bluemantle, Rouge Dragon, and Portcullis. The Earl Marshall is the Duke of Norfolk, and he is the head of the College of Arms.

TIMES FACTS

Two-fifths of the matter of the 'Times' is frequently unwritten at seven o'clock in the evening, and before the next morning the paper has to be set up, stereotyped, and printed. Each day's impression contains more than a million pieces of type, and there are generally seventy-two columns, or 17,500 lines. It employs 110 compositors and twenty-five pressmen, and is printed on the Walter Press from a continuous roll of paper over three miles long, at the rate of 100 copies per minute for each machine.

ALL AT SEA

NAUTICAL TERMS

Keel-hauling was a punishment in the Dutch navy – sometimes facetiously termed 'undergoing a great hardship.' It consisted in suspending a man with a weight at his feet from a rope rove through a block on the fore-yardarm, and with another rope attached to his legs and passed under the keel and up to the opposite fore-yardarm, drawing him into the water and under the bottom to the other side.

The 'loth to depart' was the signal sounded on outward-bound men-o'-war for visitors to leave the ship.

The pamban-manche is the snake-boat of Cochin China, a double-banked canoe some sixty feet long, paddled by a score of men, and frequently attaining a speed of twelve miles an hour.

The chess-trees are a piece of oak or other hard wood bolted to the top sides of a ship before the gangway for hauling the main tack down to. The trestle-trees are two pieces of hard wood standing fore and aft on the hounds. The cross-trees are two pieces of hard wood which stand athwart ships on scores cut into the trestle-trees; the tops, when present, are rested on the cross-trees. The spirketting is the strake of planks immediately over the waterway, extending up so as to form the lower sill of the port. The stemson is a large arching piece of compass timber, bolted inside of the apron to the stem. The sternson is a knee-piece of oak scarphed into the keelson and fayed into the throats of the transoms. The keelson is an inner keel laid along the middle of the floor timbers.

The lightest boat is the dingey, which is fourteen feet long; the jolly-boat comes next, say it is eighteen feet long; then the gig, say twenty-four feet long; then the cutter, say twenty-eight feet long; then the galley, say thirty-two feet long; then the pinnace, of the same length; and then the launch, say forty feet long.

BELLS AT SEA

A bell means a half-hour. There are seven 'watches' (not time-pieces, but divisions of the twenty-four hours). There are the afternoon watch, from noon to 4 p.m.; the first dog-watch, from 4 p.m. to 6 p.m.; the second dog, from 6 p.m. to 8 p.m.; the first watch, from 8 p.m. to midnight; the middle watch, from midnight to 4 a.m.; the morning watch, from 4 a.m. to 8 a.m.; and the forenoon watch, from 8 a.m. to noon. The dog watches are introduced so as to prevent the men being on duty during the same hours on two consecutive days, as they would be were all the watches four hours long. At the end of the first half-hour of each watch the bell is struck once, at the end of the second half-hour twice, and so on. One bell therefore denotes 12.30, 4.30, 8.30 a.m. or p.m., or 6.30 p.m. Two bells denote 1, 5, or 9 a.m. or p.m. Three bells 7.30 p.m., or 1.30, 5.30, or 9.30 a.m. or p.m. Four bells show 2, 6, and 10 a.m. or p.m. Five bells 2.30, 6.30, and 10.30 a.m. or p.m. Six bells 3, 7, and 11 a.m. or p.m. Seven bells 3.30, 7.30, 11.30 a.m. or p.m. Eight bells noon or midnight, or 8 or 4 o'clock in the night or in the morning.

LEFT AND RIGHT AT SEA

Larboard and starboard are the two Italian phrases *quello bordo* – that side, and *questo bordo* – this side, contracted first into '*lo bordo* and *sto bordo*, and then into *larboard* and *starboard.*

SAFETY AT SEA

The rhymed rule of the road at sea was written by Thomas Gray – no relation to the 'Elegy' man. It is in all the signal-books. The following is the official version:

> When both side lights you see ahead,
> Port your helm and show your red,
> Green to green, or red to red,
> Perfect safety, go ahead!
> If to your starboard red appear,
> It is your duty to keep clear,
> To act as judgment says is proper,
> To port or starboard, back or stop her.
> But when upon your port is seen
> A steamer's starboard light of green,
> There's not so much for you to do,
> For green to port keeps clear of you.
> Both in safety and in doubt,
> Always keep a good look-out;
> In danger, with no room to turn,
> Ease her! stop her! go astern!

MAIL STEAMER CREW

The staff of an Indian mail steamer may be taken as consisting of a commander, five officers, a surgeon, a carpenter, a boatswain, three quartermasters, six engineers, a purser, clerk, head steward, twenty-two stewards, two stewardesses, cook, baker, butcher, pantryman, storekeeper, and barman. All these would be Europeans, and the natives would number about one hundred and twenty-six, forty-three of them being lascars, and forty-nine coal-trimmers.

ARTS AND LETTERS

FIDDLESTICKS

Fiddle is not 'a vulgar word.' It is of the same ancestry as 'violin,' and of a better strain. Thus *fides* is Latin for string, *fidicula* is its diminutive, 'a little string.' *Fidicula* in the Low Latin becomes *fidula*, which in Italian was softened in to viola, of which the diminutive is violino, and the English adaptation violin. But fiddle is of much more direct parentage. *Fidicula* became *fideille* in old French, and *fideille* became in old English *fidel*, which in modern English changed its spelling into fiddle. Fiddle was *fithele* in Anglo-Saxon, *fithel* in Scottish, *fiedel* in High German, and *vedel* in Low German. It is worth noting that the Italian diminutive is 'ino,' while the augmentative is 'one,' whence violino, the little viol, violone, the big viola, and violoncello, the little-big viola!

WILLOW PATTERN

The mandarin had a daughter, who fell in love with his secretary, who lived on the island at the top of the plate. The father overheard them whispering under the orange-tree, and forbade their marriage. The lovers eloped, and hid in the gardener's cottage, and then escaped in a boat to the island. The mandarin pursued them, and would have flogged them to death, when lo! they were transformed into the pair of turtle-doves you see in the sky. The mandarin, with his whip, and the secretary and his bride, with the distaff, are on the bridge. The two-storey house is the mandarin's; inside the fence there is an orange-tree, also a peach-tree. The willow is at the end of the bridge. The gardener's cottage has the worst garden round it.

SHAKESPEARE

The name is generally spelt Shakespeare, but you can take your choice, as there are four thousand ways of spelling the name according to English orthography. Here are a few of the four thousand, as appearing in old documents – Shakspere, Shaxpere, Shakspire, Shaxspere, Schaksper, Shakespere, Shakespeare, Schakespeyr, Shaxespeare, Shagspere, Shaxpur, Shaxsper, Shaksper, Shackspeare, Saxpere, Shakespire, Shakespeire, Shackespeare, Shakaspear, Shaxper, Shakespear, Shaxpeare, Shakspeere, Shaxbure, Shackspeyr, Shakespear, Schakesper, etc., etc.

BAD SPELLER

We do not know who is the worst-educated speller, but there is an oft-quoted letter of the Duchess of Norfolk to Cromwell, Earl of Essex, which will give you some idea of aristocratic orthography in the sixteenth century. The Duchess wishes to write, 'My very good lord – Here I send you in token of the new year a glass of setyll set in silver gilt; I pray you take it in worth. An I were able it should be better. I would it were worth a thousand crowns.' What she does write is, 'My ffary gode lord – her I sand you in tokyn hoff the neweyer a glasse hoff setyl set in sellfer gyld. I pra you tak hit in wort. An hy wer habel het shoulde be bater. I woll hit was wort a M crone.' From which it is apparent that her grace spoke with what we should now call a strong rustic burr, and was very liberal with poor letter h. The language changes, the pronunciation changes, with every generation, and even the spelling differs with the age. Notwithstanding her seemingly absurd orthography, the Duchess, for her time, was probably better educated than you are.

ODE TO TEA

The conceit is Waller's. It occurs in a sonnet dedicated to Queen Catherine of Braganza, who had expressed her royal pleasure at the flavour of a cup of tea. Here it is. You may find it useful to wind up a speech in your next temperance debate:-

> Venus her myrtle, Phoebus has his bays;
> Tea both excels, which she vouchsafes to praise.
> The best of queens, and best of herbs we owe
> To that bold nation which the way did show
> To the fair region where the sun does rise
> Whose rich productions we so justly prize.
> The Muse's friend, tea does our fancy aid,
> Repress those vapours which the head invade,
> And keeps that palace of the soul serene,
> Fit on her birthday to salute the Queen.

✳

Chapter 7

'ABOUT FOOTBALL AND OTHER BALLS'

Manly sports for boys

THIS chapter title is taken from the first volume of the B.O.P., page 259, if you want to check. Sporting activities, from cricket to football to rowing to athletics to cycling to lacrosse, were well-covered in the BOY'S OWN PAPER, with much coverage of home teams and visitors, usually from the colonies, and

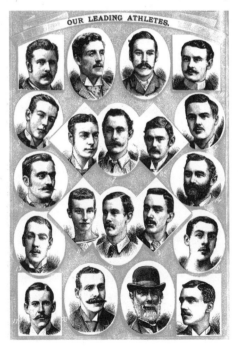

almost without exception sporting large amounts of facial hair and the occasional bowler hat.

The sports articles were extremely popular with the B.O.P.'s readers, but the problem with having a magazine that seemed to address precisely the topics that were your personal passion was that you could never get enough of the articles that interested you:

Before you write long melancholy letters, complaining that such and such a sport has 'never been touched upon,' you might take the trouble to consult the indexes and make sure that you are right. Swimming has already been dealt with, and quite a famous lot of articles were devoted to it in our first volume; the whole summer of 1881 was taken up with a well-known series of practical cricket papers; and 'the dear old Rugby game you never mention' formed a prominent feature of the paper all through last winter. The only way in which we could oblige one young gentleman would be by making every weekly number consist of a combination of itself and every other weekly number which has preceded it – give him, in fact, a real good pennyworth of some three thousand pages!

– oOo –

We knew the station of our readers, but we were not aware that bicycling was the sport of the poor and football that of the rich. We gave ten consecutive articles on bicycling in our second volume – long after you say you began to take in the BOY'S OWN PAPER – and at present we can do no more. To one boy who can ride a bicycle there are at least a dozen who can and do play football, but even if it were not so each sport and pastime must have its place. With regard to canoe-building, we are again unable to agree with you. A canoe costs no more than a decent bicycle; boys can and do make canoes – they cannot make bicycles; all they can do is to buy the different parts ready finished and screw them together. The finished materials of a bicycle cost more than those of a canoe, as also do the raw materials. In short, we think your letter a very foolish one from beginning to end, and only notice it to give you a chance of your seeing the absurdity of your silly selfishness. You will find it safer through life never to despise your fellows' amusements – nor their abilities.

Accounts of the 1884 Boat Race or football season can be somewhat arid from a twenty-first century perspective. The occasional nuggets of interesting writing in the articles deal with more unusual sports and pastimes.

Not surprisingly, baseball, because of the B.O.P.'s abhorrence of anything American, is described as 'rounders made wearisome,' but the paper has more time for lacrosse perhaps because its North American origins gave it a tinge of that exoticism that is conveyed so well in the poem in Chapter 4, page 96, *There Once was a Funny Old Sioux.*

When Lacrosse was first played must always remain a mere matter of conjecture. Its origin is undoubtedly due to the barbarous race who inhabited the American continent at the time of its discovery. Some writers have endeavoured, not without considerable skill, to impart to it the odour of centuries. Lacrosse is certainly the sport of the Redskins, although we have no information as to its earliest appearance among them....

The Indian of North America is commonly supposed to be a grim and sober creature, who never laughs, a man who at all times conducts himself in a sedate and rather gloomy manner. He is very dignified and never smiles. It is said that when at home he is always thinking of the war-path, or planning a grand and mighty hunt, or sitting by his wigwam thinking of nothing in particular. Now, as a matter of fact, the Indian has been strangely misrepresented. It has been discovered that he really liked a little fun, and could enjoy a game as well as any one.

Just in case this outburst of tolerance and understanding was going too far, the article went on to describe an England tour of a Canadian Indian lacrosse team and made fun of their names:

Our readers may gather some amusement from the names of the Indians, which were as follows: –

Teir Karoniare, or Blue Spotted.
Aton8a Tekanennao8iheu, or Hickory Wood Split.
Sha8atis Anasotako, or Pick the Feather.

Sha8atis Aientonni, or Hole in the Sky.
8ishe Taiennontii, or Flying Mane.
Aton8a Teronko8a, or The Loon.
8ishe Ononsanoron, or Deer House.
Saksarii Tontariiakan, or Crossing the River.
Tier Skanenrati, or Outside the Multitude.
Rasar Kanentakeron, or Scattered Branches.
Kor Kanentakeron, or Spruce Branches.
Saksarii Shakosennakete, or Great Arm.
Alon8a Ton8nnata, or Wild Wind.

Rasar Kanentakeron was a great chief in his own country, and acted as captain of the team.

Nowhere in this particular article was any information given about the scores on the tour – perhaps the team beat the British hollow – but the important matters *were* reported:

> Her Majesty the Queen was gracious enough to command the appearance of the teams at Windsor, and was so pleased with the game as to remain a spectator much longer than had been anticipated. [*It is not clear whether this means five minutes instead of three, or an hour rather than twenty minutes.*]

Another funny foreigner reported on in the B.O.P.'s sporting columns was the Sultan of Morocco:

> NOTWITHSTANDING that Morocco has not yet emerged from that state of barbarism in which public roads are unknown, the pursuit of cycling appears to have been taken up with much enthusiasm by the Sultan of those dominions. Mr. Howarth gives a curious account in the 'Bicycling News' of his Majesty's achievement, upon a track which he has had specially laid down in the gardens of his palace. At first he rode a single tricycle under the tuition of the English officer who holds the chief

military command in Morocco. Soon, however, he tired of the task of working the pedals, as also, perhaps, of the falls which he encountered in riding too near the edge of the gardens, which are unprotected by any wall or parapet. A brilliant idea then occurred to him. He had a large velocipede constructed which could be driven by slave labour. In the centre is a handsome embossed couch with gold and silver drapery, upon which he sits like a good Moor, cross-legged. Overhead is an umbrella, or imperial canopy, furnished with side curtains of crimson silk, and enriched with fringes of gold. The most characteristic things among the other fittings of this strange machine are a clock and a magnetic compass fitted upon two brackets, the one on the right and the other on the left of the seat. The Mohammedan must allow nothing to interfere with the strict observance of the hours of prayer, and in case the rider upon the tricycle is out of hearing of the proclamation of the mouddhen from the mosque tower, he is enabled with this clock and compass to ascertain the time of day and also the direction in which the devotions of the faithful are to be addressed. Latterly the tricycle has been worked by the ladies of the palace, although it is pointed out that as Moorish women are prized not so much for their beauty as for their weight, the new condition is not favourable to speed. The Sultan is described as in the prime of life, just turned forty years of age, and of the best Moorish type, fair-skinned, dark haired, and comely featured.

The serious, manly sport of *English* cycling in the 19th century, to the modern eye at least, seems just as amusing as a cycling Sultan. Bike design had not settled into the familiar 'handlebars-and-two-wheels' of today, and the array of ironmongery that could be seen on the streets of English towns defied classification or even uprightness, by the look of some of the pictures:

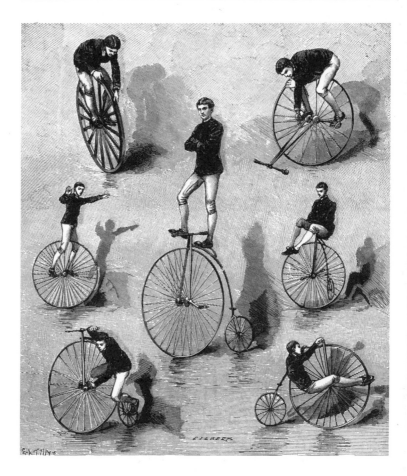

(I'm sure the man in the middle is just boasting.)

Among the sporting queries sent to the *Correspondence* column, the majority were about cricket, perhaps because it was a 'toff's' sport, and rugby was in its infancy. It was only eight years before the B.O.P. was first published that a rugby football union was formed, whereas cricket had been played in England in the 17th and 18th centuries. The BOY'S OWN PAPER published an article about a cricketing poet who flourished in the mid-18th century:

> The plain of Troy and the cricket-field have not many points in common, but each can at least boast of its heroes and its epic poet. It is true that the name of Homer is more familiar to the world than that of Mr. James Love, *alias* Dance, but, on the other hand, the personal identity of the latter is unquestionable, while considerable doubts have been expressed whether Homer ever had any real existence. If he had his blindness would have incapacitated him from cricket, and thus placed him in a lower position in the athletic world than Mr. Love attained. We need not, therefore, grudge him his poetical pre-eminence.
>
> ... He [Love] republished his poem on 'Cricket' in 1770, and we may perhaps infer its popularity from the fact that the British Museum Library contains only a single copy of the later edition and none whatever of the former.
>
> The [Richmond Cricket Ground] was thronged by enthusiastic spectators when, as on the occasion which inspired the poet, a good match was to be played, and betting on the result was far more general than, happily, is now the case. A note tells us that 'the robust cricketer plays in his shirt. The Rev. Mr. W---d particularly appears almost naked ...' and the present writer (albeit only in mid-life) can remember the time when 'flannels' were less the rule than was the chimney-pot hat ...
>
> The epic opens in a truly classical style:
>
> > 'The stumps are pitch'd. Each hero now is seen;
> > Springs o'er the fence, and bounds along the green,
> > In decent white most gracefully arrayed.
> > Each strong-built limb in all its pride display'd."

By the time of the B.O.P., naked cricketing wearing only a chimney-pot hat was frowned on, and one article gave more up-to-date sartorial advice to the would-be cricketer:

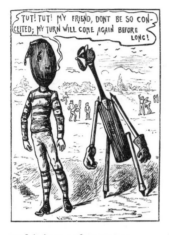

Now, taking it for granted that you, like all healthy young Englishmen, have a tub every morning, let me address you as you are standing in the buff rubbing yourself down with a rough towel. I am assuming that you are going to play in a match, and I will tell you what to eat and what to avoid, and wherewithal you should be clothed. And the last is the first necessity, as you are in the buff, and it is usual to put on your clothes before breakfast; and the third caution, as to what to avoid, comes at the same time as the last. Avoid uniforms and 'loud' dress of all kinds. Common sense and good taste are bringing men back to better ways, and they begin to find out that Harlequin shirts and thunder-and-lightning jackets could only have been invented for the benefits of tailors and haberdashers.

A high proportion of letters about sport to the B.O.P. seemed to be seeking clarification of the rules of cricket, often, it seems, to settle an argument or extract support for a challenge to an umpire's decision. The Editor's replies did not always take the query seriously:

'In cricket, when the ball is delivered, is the batsman bound to remove his bat?' There is no law that says so. He can stand stock still like an imbecile if he likes, and he will find it will greatly increase the effect if he sticks himself right in front of the wicket and shuts both eyes.

– oOo –

There is no rule against a man spoiling his bat or getting out as quickly as he likes. Should the bat not be yours the owner will probably feel himself aggrieved at your using the wrong side, but your opponents will be delighted!

– oOo –

A BOY WITH ONE LEG ONLY – You were out. The ball was caught before it touched the ground. It matters not how many fielders may have tried at it and touched it with their fingers' ends.

– oOo –

There is nothing 'knotty,' as some of you phrase it, about any of your questions. If a man runs out of his ground, and the wicket is put down, he is out; if the players have crossed, the one who runs for the wicket that is put down is out; if the wicket is put down to which the man is running, and from which the other man has not stirred, no one is out. If a ball pitches anyhow or anywhere between the wickets, and is properly bowled in other respects, it is not a 'no ball.' If a wicket-keeper puts his hands in front of the wicket, and the stump is touched by the ball, the man is not out – the wicket-keeper's hands must be behind the wicket until the ball has

passed it. And so on, and so on. There is not a question raised by any one of you that has not been fully answered in Dr. Grace's articles, and for the future we must refer you to them, and only answer such queries as have not been previously dealt with.

– oOo –

SOME IGNORANT CRICKETERS should have read the laws of cricket, which they cannot have done at present. It is almost inconceivable how they could imagine such a thing. How can a man be run out if his wicket is not put down? and how can it be *his* wicket if it is *somebody else's*?

– oOo –

If a batsman is out, he is out, no matter how many people say so. But if the fieldsmen yell and shout 'out' before the ball has reached him he is decidedly not out, as such a proceeding is manifestly unfair.

– oOo –

Oh! why, and oh! why? Cricket Law No. 10: 'The ball must be bowled; if thrown or jerked, the umpire shall call no-ball.' Cricket

Law No. 11: 'The bowler shall deliver the ball with one foot on the ground behind the bowling-crease, and within the return-crease, otherwise the umpire shall call no-ball.' There is no other no-ball. Why should you invent one? What is there to trouble an umpire? It is not the M.C.C. that is to blame, but your own stupidity.

– oOo –

What do you mean by 'accidentally'? Where is the umpire to draw the line? If the ball is touched by the hands the penalty must be enforced.

– oOo –

The 'Laws of Cricket' are not likely to deal with such an absurdity. If you like to hold your bat with both hands behind it, pray do – and get out. You will be a most popular cricketer – with your opponents.

– oOo –

There are quite ways enough at present for getting a batsman out without inventing new ones. Why not read the laws? If the matter be not mentioned therein, you are simply wasting time in asking the question. In what law of cricket does it say that the striker is out if he pick up the bail which has been knocked off? In what law does it say he is out if he hits the ball with the 'hedge of his bat'? We fear that your umpire must be out – of his mind.

– oOo –

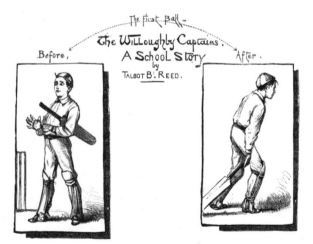

The First Ball –
The Willoughby Captains:
A School Story
by
Talbot B. Reed.

Before,   After.

A man cannot be caught out off a no-ball. As a case in point, Mr. A.P. Lucas, in the M.C.C. match against the Australians last July, deliberately slogged at a no-ball bowled by Spofforth, and was caught at mid-on by Giffen, but continued his innings as though nothing had happened, to the wonderment of not a few of the onlookers.

– oOo –

A CORRESPONDENT whose signature we are not quite sure about, says: 'The other day, while playing a side with the boys, I chanced to bowl a ball which knocked the off and leg stumps out of the ground, leaving the centre wicket standing in its usual position. Can any of your cricketer friends solve the problem?' This fairly beats us, though optical delusions of a somewhat similar nature have been produced before now by very smart wicket-keepers.

– oOo –

Here is another curiosity. 'A match was played on Ascot Racecourse.

One of the batsmen drove the ball in amongst the crowd, when a large dog seized the ball, grasping it tightly. Were the fielders right in calling 'Lost ball!' or the batsmen justified in running until the ball was returned, as the dog held the ball firmly in his mouth?' Here the batsmen could have kept on running, if it amused them, but they should clearly only have scored for the lost ball. So long as you cannot get at it, the ball must be held to be lost, and it does not matter if you know where it is. There is an old story of an Irish sailor who dropped a kettle overboard which bears somewhat on this point. He went to his captain, and inquired if a thing could be lost if he knew where it was. 'Surely not,' said the captain. 'Thin bedad, sorr,' quoth Pat, 'your kettle isn't lost at all, at all, for it's at the bottom of the say!'

– oOo –

'Is a man out when the ball twists in from behind the wicket?' Did you ever see a ball twist in that way? – a boomerang might, but a ball!

Queries about sporting records in different sports were also popular in pre-*Guinness Book of Records* days, although a hundred and twenty years on, the figures given convey the impression that athletes and sportsmen conducted their business at a snail's pace:

We are not quite clear as to your meaning, but the fastest amateur time for one mile is 4 min. 23 1/5 sec., and the race in which it was made has been described in these pages. The thousand yards has been run in 2 min. 20 4/5 sec., but there is no record for five hundred yards. The quarter-mile has been done in 50 2/5 sec.

– o O o –

The quickest cricket scoring on record occurred in a match played last Easter Monday between the James Thorne and Thornbury Clubs at Alveston, in Gloucestershire. James Thorne went in first, and were all out at a quarter past one for 42. Thornbury then commenced their innings, and at ten minutes past two an hour's adjournment took place for lunch. Stumps were drawn at twenty-five minutes past six, and Thornbury had lost only three wickets for 674 runs, or at the rate of 162 runs per hour! Dr. E. M. Grace got 228, Dr. W.G. Grace not out 196, and Mr. J. Cranston not out 174.

– o O o –

You must have very queer ideas as to what constitutes a 'Best on Record' to suppose that a private note to an editor would be sufficient testimony. If your friend can run the quarter-mile in less time than any one else, let him do it under proper arrangements on some well-known ground, and then, when it is accepted by everybody else, we will notice his performance – and not before.

– o O o –

The quickest hundred yards in a bath was swum by E.T. Jones, of Leeds, in 1 min. 8 1/2 sec. at Lambeth; in still water by W. Cole in 1 min. 15 1/2 sec. in the Serpentine.

– o O o –

The best throw of the cricket-ball recorded is that by G. Brown in 1819, on Wolverton Common, when he is said to have thrown it one hundred and thirty-seven yards, but it is the custom to doubt the measurement. W.F. Forbes threw one hundred and thirty-two yards at Oxford in 1876. A hundred yards is a good throw.

– o O o –

The greatest distance ever run in one hour is eleven miles nine hundred and seventy yards, by L. Bennett, professional, at Lillie Bridge on 3 April 1863.

– oOo –

William Gale's two feats were walking 1,500 miles in 1,000 hours – that is, beginning to walk at the stroke of each hour, and after he had completed a mile and a half resting till the next hour – and walking 4,000 quarter-miles in 4,000 periods of ten minutes each – that is, walking a quarter of a mile and then resting until the ten minutes had expired.

– oOo –

The longest running hop-step-and-jump was done by R. Knox, of Newstead, on Leith Links, in August 1870. He covered 47ft. 7in. We do not know the longest running wide jump in Scotland; but J. Howard, of Bradford, is said to have cleared 29ft. 7in. in May 1854, on Chester racecourse. He had a 5lb. dumb-bell in each hand, and took off from a wedge-shaped block of wood. The widest recorded horse-jump is that made by Chandler, who, ridden by Captain Broadley, cleared 37ft. in a steeplechase at Warwick on 22 March 1847.

– oOo –

There is no difficulty; 'the lowest score in a cricket match in a single innings made by a club' was 0.

– oOo –

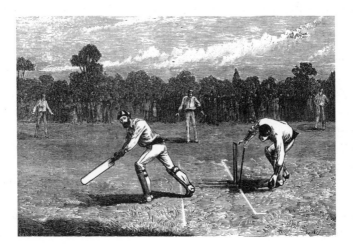

Such things are not recorded. We once saw E. M. Grace hit an eight for Lansdown against Marlborough College, and have read of the Hon. F. Ponsonby hitting a nine at Parker's Piece, but bigger hits than these have probably been made in country clubs. In most cricketing villages there is a legend of some slogging blacksmith or butcher who once made a wondrous hit.... The heaviest scoring in a first-class match that we remember at the present moment was on 19, 20 and 21 June 1876, at Prince's. The match was Middlesex v. Oxford University, and in it 551 overs were bowled. Mr. I.D. Walker made 110, Mr. W.H. Game 141, Mr. A. Burghes 104. The elevens made innings of 612, 439, and 166 for four wickets, so that 1,217 runs were scored, and only twenty-four wickets fell. The highest score in an innings was 742, made by East Melbourne v. Tasmania, on 6, 7 and 8 December 1879.

For the rest of the queries, there was no knowing what boys would ask:

Jaques, of Hatton Garden, is the manufacturer of the game of squails, and he would tell you all about them.

– oOo –

As you do not say where you hail from, it is impossible for us to tell you of a neighbouring cricket-ground.

– oOo –

We have nothing to add to our article on training. You should not over-fatigue yourself. Try ten miles. When you can finish that without tiring, try twelve miles, and so on. There is no object in making a toil of a pleasure to the extent you say you do.

– oOo –

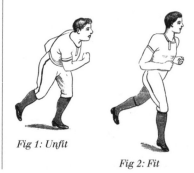

Fig 1: Unfit

Fig 2: Fit

Commence your letter 'Sir' – never say 'Hon. Sir' – and consult our articles on Cricket, by Dr. W.G. Grace. Nothing better (or fuller) on the practical part of the game has yet been written.

– oOo –

Here is what TOODLES says about Knucklebones, and an uncommonly interesting game we should think it was! 'Order of Knucklebones Practice, ones, twos, threes, fours, creepmouse, chuckups, dux 1, dux 2, dux 3, dux 4, clicks, non-clicks, postman's-knock, double postman's-knock, fingers, inches, spances, short arms, long arms, and triangles; squares, daggers, swords; pockets 1, pockets 2, pockets 3, pockets 4, everlastings!' F.J. BUCKELL says that the game is identical with Dibs, played with five small bones from the knuckles of a sheep, and is treated of in Hoyle. In a recent B.O.P it was pretty fully described.

– oOo –

How to become an acrobat? Give up the idea altogether. You are too old, and, by the time you see this, you will have become too sensible. How many postage stamps are there in the world? Here also the progress of time will have rendered our research unnecessary.

– oOo –

Expert skaters can cut their names on the ice just as you can write your name without taking your pen off the paper; and, as in your case, the performance is not always much of a success.

– oOo –

We have no preference for Rugby over Association Football. We described the Rugby game first for two reasons – one, that it is the oldest game; the other, that, taking the whole kingdom, it is the most played. Association Football will be treated of at length in another volume. We cannot give everything at once.

– oOo –

All in good time; every sport we have will in its turn be treated of by the highest living authority on it we can find. Cricket, for instance, was done by Dr. W.G. Grace; Rugby Football by Dr. Bell Irvine; and the others will follow in due course.

– oOo –

INTENDING TRICYCLER – See our article on Tricycles last August. The machine you mention is the 'Otto.' Accidents can occur with tricycles just as they can with anything else in this world. We do not see anything specially dangerous about them. They are certainly safer than bicycles.

– o O o –

We do not think thirty miles too much for a day's walk; many greater distances are frequently done by healthy young men. A walking-tour at such a rate, however, means merely walking for walking's sake, and the neglect of everything of interest on the road.

– o O o –

It is not customary in England to fill footballs with gas, whatever it may be in Belgium. There is just a chance that the lifting power would be so very much improved that a kick-off would send the ball aloft, and leave it there like a balloon.

– o O o –

Alas! too curious youth! 'What an acrobat does to acquire the means of his twisting his legs about, such as putting them round his neck, or if he apply any lotion, oil, etc., to the joints?' We must not divulge trade secrets, but we have been told that he eats nothing but tire cement, and enjoys a daily application of strap oil!

– o O o –

Yours is by no means a solitary case, as we get letters from New Zealand by almost every mail, Pacific and direct. No interest is taken in this country in wire-walking except by professional acrobats, and an article on the subject would be of slender interest, and likely to lead to protests against our encouraging Blondinism, which is of no practical use in athletics. 'Dought' is a queer way of spelling doubt.

– o O o –

Depends not a little on circumstances. For all kinds of outdoor sports, and most kinds of hard manual work, the belt would undoubtedly have the advantage; yet, to some weakly backs and drooping shoulders, as well as in some sedentary occupations, braces are found to afford a measure of support.

– o O o –

We do not think you could stand a walking tour in your present condition. If you try, ten miles a day will be enough.

– o O o –

No boy should ride till fifteen; and then the machine ought to be proportioned to his weight. If not, he will suffer in after-life.

– o O o –

Nearly every cricketer has heard of E.H. Budd. He was a very famous player, and is over and over again mentioned in all the principal books, but he was not the 'greatest player in England.' Cricket reputations are at the best ephemeral, and good players have been so numerous that it is no disgrace not to remember them all.

– o O o –

What a queer lot of cricketers your friends must be! 1. The captain of an eleven has the management of the match for his side, and what he decides to do the other players should acquiesce in. The umpires can be changed under certain circumstances (see XLIII of the Cricket Laws). 2. You are not generally supposed to play cricket with cheats, and the sooner you cease your acquaintance with the so remarkably clever captains you mention the better. 3. If a batsman hits a ball with the wrong side, or edge, of the bat, he is not thereby out, but we should think he soon would be from other causes.

– o O o –

If the balls are the same size and weight as the brass ones you will do no harm; but if those you have are much lighter than the others your hands will be puzzled when you try the heavier ones. There is no reason why you should not retain the wood; cover it with gold paper, and it will look just as well.

– o O o –

When you are on a bicycle you will find it the best plan to give vehicles a wide berth. You may have certain rights of the road, but it is much the safest to get out of the way. As your vehicle is supposed to be under more control than that drawn by a horse, you are expected as a matter of courtesy to give way – just as a rowing boat has to give way to a sailing boat. 2. Your armpit is under your arm; your shoulder is over your arm.

– o O o –

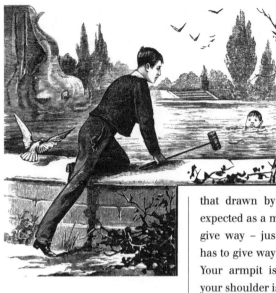

You tell us a sad tale. There seems little doubt that the poor boy had remained much too long in the water. You say that 'he gave one or two screams,' flung up his arms, and sank. To us, the symptoms look like those of a fit, and not cramp; and even in the worst cases of cramp, the sufferer can call for help instead of screaming. Even had it been a fit, it seems to have been either brought on or hastened by too long immersion.

– oOo –

When you are on a bicycle you will find it the best plan to give vehicles a wide berth. You may have certain rights of the road, but it is much the safest to get out of the way. As your vehicle is supposed to be under more control than that drawn by a horse, you are expected as a matter of courtesy to give way – just as a rowing boat has to give way to a sailing boat. 2. Your armpit is under your arm; your shoulder is over your arm.

– oOo –

No one can ride like a monkey for a long time without seriously injuring himself.

– oOo –

We are extremely sorry that you are at such 'a loss to find why we don't reply to your queries in our notes,' but if you will read the articles on Cricket a little more carefully you will find that questions 1, 2, 5, and 6 were therein fully answered; and of your other two questions, No. 3 is only a vulgar expression, and refers to no particular variety, its meaning being different in different districts; and No.4 is simply idiotic. Ask Alfred Shaw if he can bowl a straight ball! By the way, in your excitement, you have made rare use of poor letter *h*.

– oOo –

Slender bamboos make the best of arrows, if they are straight and have the joints sandpapered down.

Point them with ferrules. You may have to use deal for the feather end. No arrow will fly straight unless it is feathered, except by accident. Your best plan would be to buy an arrow from, say Aldred, 258, Oxford Street, W., and copy it as well as you can. We do not consider 'four golds in succession at five yards' a very remarkable performance, unless the target was microscopic.

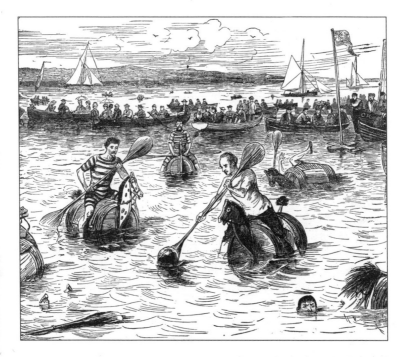

═══════════ ⟩⟨ ═══════════

Chapter 8

'A MERCIFUL MAN IS MERCIFUL TO HIS MOUSE'

Boys' pets in sickness and health

JUDGING by the columns of *Correspondence* in the BOY'S OWN PAPER, the small caged animal population of Great Britain in the late 19th century may well have exceeded the human population. The passion for pets among boys was huge and there seemed no creature that could not be domesticated to provide hours of fun for its owner.

An article called *Sea Anemones as Pets* had some good advice:

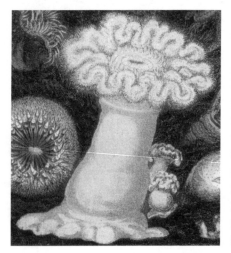

The anemones will require *feeding* at intervals, for their owner must remember that they are *animals* not *flowers*, though many people who know nothing of them think they are the latter when first seen expanded. For the first few days after they are taken from the rocks they will very likely not eat anything offered them; but when they have been deprived of their natural sustenance for a few days they will eat a tolerable number of small pieces of raw meat if allowed to fall on their expanded discs. Any pieces not eaten, and rejected portions of digested meat, must be at once taken out of the water, and any anemones that happen to die must also be removed at once, for if putrefaction once sets in the whole stock will die in a few hours.

In the monthly column *Doings for the Month* there were regular accounts of tasks to be done for some of the most frequently-kept pets. For November 1888, the column starts with GOATS – 'Nanny gives us milk, and she gives us kids, and when dead we have her head to stuff ...' [*More about stuffing later*]; then THE POULTRY RUN – after forecasting a snowy winter, the writer, probably Gordon Stables, says 'We saw last year a hen-house which permitted the snow to sift in in several directions. The owner said he never could get his fowls to lay in winter. No wonder! That young man did not deserve a new-laid egg for breakfast.'; THE PIGEON LOFT – 'We hope you have been reading up some book about your pets. You may not be able to buy, but if you are a good and earnest lad a pigeon-fancying neighbour could lend you one...'; THE AVIARY , THE RABBITRY, and THE KENNEL, and then THE BEE WORLD where 'all is quiet.'

In addition to the monthly notes, there were many long and detailed articles about individual pets. THE BOY'S OWN CAVIARY was about 'our funny wee friends the cavies'. Other articles included SNAILS AS PETS, MONKEYS AS PETS OR OTHERWISE, and, presumably for very wealthy boys, HOW TO BUY A MENAGERIE.

With this richness of choice, the first question was what to have and where to get it:

For a pet indoors, have a cat, and be kind to it. For outdoors nothing, perhaps, can equal an Abyssinian guinea-pig.

– o O o –

HEDGEHOGS – They don't do well for pets, they are as miserable in captivity as Captain Dreyfus was. Why do you write in pencil?

– o O o –

Mr. Jamrach, of St. George's Street, E., will supply you with any number of monkeys you require.

– o O o –

You can get almost any animal on earth by return of post from William Cross, 18, Earle Street, Liverpool.

It is a bad time of year for buying alligators ...

– o O o –

TORTOISES – Write to E. Sumner, 135 Oxford Street, London. He has lots of them.

– o O o –

The only 'pretty' dog that will fulfil all your requirements as to keeping quiet, giving no trouble, doing no damage, costing little to keep, etc., etc., is a crockery pug, which you can get at the nearest china shop. That will keep quite quiet, be quite clean, and cost you – nothing.

– o O o –

From the answers to queries about mice, it is clear that they were somewhat of a favourite, at least with Gordon Stables:

Dr. Stables says he has been waiting for months for such a query as yours, and is glad it has come at last. He made no mention of the dry-feeding system for mice in his paper; he kept that to himself, because he considers it both 'a lazy and a cruel plan.' But being now asked the question so directly, he replies, that in shops and places where mice are sold, they are often fed almost exclusively on canary and millet seeds, and get no moisture. This he confesses *does* keep down the smell to a large extent; but he adds, 'a merciful man is merciful to his mouse,' and still advocates the giving of stale bread and a little milk, and perfect cleanliness – a good bed and plenty of sawdust.

– o O o –

We will not forget white mice when a favourable opportunity occurs.

– o O o –

A FRIEND OF MICE – No, not a separate cage, but a large roomy one, with small dark room. Study and follow nature. Keep seed tins and food tins always full and clean. You ask, 'Does the light hurt the eyes of mice?' Well, we never saw mice in a natural state wearing green spectacles.

– o O o –

Your very sensible letter on exercise for mice will receive due consideration, and will be further answered in a future number. Anyhow, go on experimenting, and let us hear from you again.

– o O o –

We should leave the mouse alone, but see that he did not want for food. 'A black-spotted mouse, that follows us from room to room, and even sits on the fender and washes its face while we are sitting by the fireside, and sings away, and will feed out of your hand,' is a treasure that when found should be made the most of.

– o O o –

It is extremely unlikely that you will make a profit out of dormice. The most profitable outdoor pets are poultry. For indoor pets canaries are about the most promising.

– o O o –

The mice are quite right in not going into your trap. Would you, now, if you were a mouse? Get a cat.

– o O o –

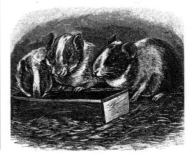

Although he had favourites, the writer of these answers came down heavily on anyone who showed signs of cruelty or neglect, whatever the creature:

No, don't cut the bird's tongue. This custom is cruel and utterly useless. Keep repeating words to it, and whistling to it. Feed it well, and it will soon imitate.

– oOo –

A boy who is so barbarous and foolish as to slit a bird's tongue ought to have his own tongue slit.

– oOo –

Certainly not. How would you like to live 'in a cellar with a small grating 3½ in wide and 9in long'?

– oOo –

Judging from your letter, we imagine that the dog's regret will not be excessive when you cease to be his master. The fact of his being 'no mortal use whatsoever' is no reason why you shouldn't pay the dog-tax, and the simple fact of your inquiring as to whether you should train him with 'kindness or cruelty' is sufficient to show that whoever trusted you with him was very ill-advised. If you cannot be kind to an animal, do not trouble yourself to keep one.

– oOo –

Your treatment altogether of your cat reads horrible. You can have no feeling in you.

– oOo –

You seem utterly ignorant in the matter of breeding. We always say it is wrong of any boy to purchase pets without having first studied their habits. Banish madness from your mind and leave the dog alone.

– oOo –

ONE BISCUIT – Yes, quite enough if you want to starve the dog to death.

– oOo –

You cruel boy, to hang your canaries in a kitchen till feathers and voice are gone! You ought to be served so yourself. Either kill them or give them different quarters, and good food with fresh water. Put them in a cheerful, sunny room.

– oOo –

ANXIOUS – wishes us to tell him a 'good way to rear a nest of young skylarks, as he has failed many times.' We reply: Leave them alone, and let the parent rear them. We decline to give any instructions for such cruelty as imprisoning skylarks in cages. You have already, by your own statement, killed many broods of skylarks. Be content with the mischief you have done, and do it no more.

For the most part, the answers address the usual kind of day to day problems that the inexperienced pet-fancier was likely to come across:

We regret to say that our education has been so neglected that we never learned how to clean hedgehogs and always left them to do it for themselves! Send us some of the insects found on them. If you keep rabbits and hedgehogs together, you may some day chance to find that the former have eaten the latter.

– o O o –

No; leave the cock bird in while the hen is sitting so long as he conducts himself like a gentleman.

– o O o –

TOBY'S PUP – We have read your long letter carefully through. Mr. Mayhew was an honest and careful writer; there is much in his book that is very good. He was also a candid man, and you will see in his preface that he says, 'The pathology of the dog is at present not properly taught, nor rightly understood, by the veterinarians who profess to alleviate canine afflictions.' But there are many errors in the work. Mayhew has

taken many of the old popular fallacies as truths – adopted them, in fact, because they seem to accord with his judgement. Well, Mr. Mayhew wrote in 1854, Dr. Gordon Stables writes in 1880; and if, as you must admit, all knowledge is progressive, and experience is constantly adding thereto, it stands to reason that 1880 must be considered more trustworthy than 1854; and of one thing we are quite convinced, namely, that if Mr. Mayhew were alive now, and revised his book, he would not

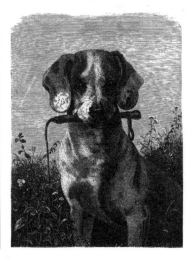

advocate filth as food, condemn a little salt in a dog's dinner, nor term a simple dose of castor-oil all but poison. Veterinary surgeons of the *new* school are far *far* different from the rough rule-of-thumb men of bygone years; but as regards the ailments of dogs, and the smaller kinds of pets, they even now do not profess to have a complete knowledge. You write well and sensibly, and we shall be glad to hear how you get on with your canine pets.

– oOo –

It is queries like yours we like to answer – practical ones. You are feeding your jay on altogether wrong principles. Do you really think that beak of his was made to eat sopped bread-and-milk? Take another look at it. The jay must smile inwardly. Give him bits of raw meat, any bone-parings from butchers, table scraps generally. He will eat anything in the shape of meat. Also gather insects for him, and garden worms, and mix for him a paste of oatmeal pretty dry. Dead mice may also be given.

– oOo –

Yes; and a hen will hatch turkey's eggs. There is nothing unusual in a cat eating kittens.

– oOo –

Yes, to all your questions. A jackdaw should have his freedom.

– oOo –

Your little bantam hen is probably a little bantam cock, and cocks do not lay. Read our article on Bantams.

– oOo –

SIX DOZEN LADY READERS – All going in for rabbits? Well, a hutch for a pair would need to be three feet by eighteen inches, and two feet high; but you must either get a book (Cassell and Co. publish one at 3s. 6d.) or read our back numbers on rabbits.

– oOo –

We may have a paper on Mule Breeding next season. It is a lengthy subject to treat here. [*This turns out to refer to canary crossbreeds, rather than the cross between an ass and a mare.*]

– oOo –

TAKING A CAT TO AMERICA – You must make friends with the cook beforehand, or one of the stewards. After you are at sea, you can let pussy have exercise.

– oOo –

FOWLS PAYING – Yes, they will pay their keep. Read our Monthly Doings.

– oOo –

PIGEON LAYING – Never mind; if she chooses to lay in a corner of the floor she will hatch there. Pigeons must be humoured.

– oOo –

FEEDING POMERANIAN, Etc – 1. On the tablescraps but give her plenty. 2. The other question is of too delicate a nature to answer. Ask any keeper.

– oOo –

Your letter arrived without the dog – at least, he was not 'annexed,' as you say. Sorry he did not come, as we are afraid we cannot help you. Your description of him as 'about 1½ feet long and about 1 foot high; long-haired, almost straight, white with a few reddish spots on the back,' is hardly precise enough for us to 'cam the breed.'

– oOo –

No, why 'should we be shocked at a girl taking in the B.O.P'? Feed your favourites on garden roots and greens, with every morning a sop of bread-and-milk. They like grains in winter.

– oOo –

You are right and wrong, and observant. Many female birds, after they have finally ceased to lay eggs, assume the plumage, voice, and general demeanour of the male. 'Crowing Hens' are familiar to all poultry keepers, and are generally slaughtered as being unlucky. The late Charles Waterton rescued one of these metamorphosed hens, and after its death stuffed it. The bird is still to be seen in Waterton's Museum at Ushaw College.

– oOo –

The bed, or sleeping-box, for your pair of rats, if 9in. by 12in., will do; and the size of the yard is fair, though it might be bigger. The swing we never tried, and do not think it would work; but you might make a pole with a spiral staircase to run up; the pole should protrude at least a foot from the top of the tower. These rodents dearly love to look about them.

INQUIRER – 'Salt cat' used in pigeonries is simply a mixture of old lime, gravel, and salt, or old lime, loam, and salt.

– o O o –

Dear boy, no: the 'salt-cat' referred to is a very innocent affair! We do *not* mean that you are to procure a pussy-cat, kill her, roast her, salt her, and hang her up in the pigeon-loft for the birds to peck at – by way of venting their spleen, I suppose you thought. For a definition of 'salt-cat,' which at best is but a vulgar word, see DOINGS FOR THE MONTH of July; but pray do not give us such a fright again. We nearly sprang bolt out of the editorial chair when we read your terrible letter.

– o O o –

C.O. desires to know 'the best way to feed a pet raven'. Give it anything that you can eat yourself. His daintiest treat, however, according to the Rev. J.G. Wood, is a large rat. 'He will,' writes Mr Wood to us, 'peck a hole in the side, eat away the whole of the soft parts, and leave the skin turned inside out. I had one for some time. He died from a surfeit of table linen.'

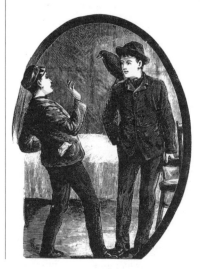

Full of veterinary wisdom as these articles were, they seem unable to prevent a dreadful toll of morbidity that dominated the *Correspondence* columns.

Without knowing how you feed and treat your canary we could not be expected to tell the reason of its being devoid of feathers round the neck. Give it plain seeds, a little green food, and a portion of ripe, sweet apple. Anoint the neck with pure salad oil.

– o O o –

The asthmatic wheeze of the canary is probably occasioned by the Red Mite. Dust the bird and cage with Hardeman's Insect Powder.

– oOo –

We do not see that you can do anything with the bird. It has got a fright, and will hardly recover it. Hang the cage in a cheerful place, feed well, and keep quiet.

Your squirrel is suffering from the effects of external parasites. Begin by putting it in a temporary cage while you thoroughly clean and disinfect the other. Scald it with boiling water ...

– oOo –

If we were to publish your 'cure for distemper' we would kill dogs by the score. Distemper has no cure. We treat symptoms and guide the canine patient through it – and nursing is half the battle.

– oOo –

As we go to press six weeks before we publish, we fear this will not reach you in time to do your canaries good. You evidently paired too soon. The weather this year was very trying, and the birds many of them weakly.

– oOo –

Your fish will never live in the wooden tank. There are other things beside the putty which will kill them.

– oOo –

The hen has bumble-foot; let out the matter with a very sharp penknife if there be any. Afterwards dress with zinc ointment; keep the foot clean, and let her wear a stocking.

– oOo –

Oil the bare places; give no hemp. You ought not to have cut the cockatoo's bill.

– oOo –

It is so unusual an accident that we could not give advice without seeing the rabbit.

– oOo –

BOY GEORGE – Kill the goldfish. Its water has been impure or badly aerated. Have you plants in your aquarium?

– oOo –

You say your pigeon was sick the other day, and want us to say what was the matter. Funny lad! Pigeons suffer from fifty ills, and you do not name a symptom.

– o O o –

Egg-eating. The radical cure is to kill the fowl. All other plans have at times failed to cure the habit – blown eggs filled with mustard and cayenne, stone eggs, etc. Do you give plenty of gravel?

– o O o –

It appears to be an aneurism. Could not say for certain without seeing it.

– o O o –

RABBIT WITH COLD – 1. Keep extra dry and warm, and give mash every night. You cannot do much more. Separate the sick from the healthy. It may be snuffles. 2. Is it your own nose or the rabbit's you refer to in your second query? You are a queer boy!

– o O o –

CANARY ASTHMATICAL – Complaint all but incurable. Feed rather better, adding a little egg and bread crumb to the diet. Often the result of weakness.

JACKDAW WITH BAD FOOT – When the matter is cleared out, dress with ointment of zinc, but keep clean.

– o O o –

MAGPIE BALD – The bird wants sunning about more ... Maggie will die if she has not more freedom, and she will be better dead.

– o O o –

CHICKENS ILL – It was not pip, but the gapes. Try Spratts remedy.

– o O o –

KITTEN ILL – It is of a weakly constitution. If still alive, give plenty of cream, fish, egg, minced raw meat, and clean water. Keep in the house at night.

– o O o –

DOG'S EYE SCRATCHED BY A CAT – It is too late now, we fear. The dog must either be better or blind. But hot fomentations was the correct treatment, and rest in a dark apartment.

– o O o –

JACKDAW ILL – He has caught cold and it has become chronic. This is the nearest we can get to it but he might have a gathering in his throat. Don't let him sleep in a draught.

– o O o –

We would not tell you if we knew. Birds have quite enemies enough without being killed wholesale by poisoned grain.

– o O o –

E. SAXBY is in grief because two turtle-doves he has 'always fight when together,' and are 'miserable apart.' They must be Irish. If a big cage and plenty to eat do not serve to mend matters, let them part to meet again never more.

– o O o –

When hens suck their own eggs the best thing you can do is kill them off.

– o O o –

RAT WITH SORES (Bobby) – We fear, Bobby, we can't help you. A rat with sores is usually a 'gone coon.' Try sulphur ointment. Keep the cage clean. [*A 'gone coon' (meaning raccoon) was the same as a 'dead duck.'*]

– o O o –

There is something radically wrong in your pigeon-loft; we cannot say what.

– o O o –

BERTIE CLERK ... will know by this time whether the squirrel is dead or alive.

The death of pets was all too common an occurrence. It was only human to ask 'Why?', although the reason was often only too apparent:

Certainly your canaries died of sunstroke. It was so foolish to hang them in the glare. We fear you are not the only foolish boy in this respect.

– o O o –

Dog will be dead ere this reaches you. You have fed him wrongly. See

Dr. Gordon Stables's articles in back numbers.

– o O o –

You mean what was the cause or nature of its illness, we suppose, since there can be no doubt as to that of its death, when you acknowledge to having drowned it.

– o O o –

Well, it was suffering from inflammation of the lungs, the result of a sudden chill probably, for it was plump, and its illness could not have been of long duration. Warmth, in a moist atmosphere, with one-drop doses of oxymel of squills three or four times a day might, in all probability, have saved it.

– oOo –

DEAD CANARY ('Mother of Four Boys') – Careful examination of this bird failed to reveal any disease. All the organs were in a healthy state, but the whole of the alimentary canal was empty; at least there were a few grains of sand in the gizzard, but no vestige of food. It is therefore certain that the bird died from starvation, how induced there is no evidence to show; but as it was extremely thin, it is probable that it had been irregularly attended to, or perhaps mice pilfered its provisions.

– oOo –

Your plan of killing rabbits is old-fashioned but good. Why we recommend the stick instead of the hand is because a mere boy would not have the strength to stun with the latter.

– oOo –

We fear, by the time you get this reply, your pigeons will be past relief. Remove them at once, if alive, to a comfortable, clean place ...

– oOo –

Your pigeon is dead by now, so we need not reply. Nursing young pigeons that go light is a thankless task.

– oOo –

Your pigeon is doubtless dead by now. 2 and 3. The troubles that afflict your pigeonry are no doubt caused by inattention to matters sanitary.

– oOo –

CHEAP PARROTS – The 10s 6d ones all die. If you trust to Cross of Liverpool, to send a really good one, he will do it, but not under 25s or 30s.

– oOo –

YOUNG TURTLE – It won't live, and is probably dead ere now.

– oOo –

We have had many cases of sickness among parrots precisely like yours, but have hitherto been very unsuccessful in our treatment. By the time this reaches you your parrot will be dead, so there is no good in advising you. But it is the change of food and climate that injures parrots. They are brought home in ship-loads, and sold cheap. Anyone buying a young parrot ought to let it have plenty of chilies at first, and a little hemp, with nuts of different kinds.

– oOo –

An ill-tempered rabbit is best out of the world.

– oOo –

Yes; they would not be poisonous, but would require to be bled at once. A smart blow behind the ear is the best way of killing them. But you should see this done before you do it yourself.

– oOo –

KILLING PIGEONS – Drawing the neck.

Finally, left with a dead pet, and a pair of idle hands, some boys thought it might be a good idea to stuff it. The B.O.P. was happy to supply instructions in an article but warned against the horrors of a botched job:

> Dogs, cats and domestic animals generally, which during their lives have been pets of the family, are usually stuffed with the view of keeping their memories green in the minds of the bereaved owners. They are accordingly set up singly, and if they are not most carefully stuffed, and managed as to attitude, they become in a few months mere caricatures of former friends, staring, dusty, deformed, and horrible. No amateur, therefore, should attempt to stuff and set up a dead favourite until he has entirely mastered the beautiful art of taxidermy. Then, if he happens to own some animal pet that he means to stuff when its short life is over, let him study the attitudes of the creature while alive, and sketch, if he can, those which are most graceful. In one of those he ought to be set up. A pet dog stuffed, for example, in a standing position is to me an abomination, and almost an insult to the canine race.

The animals which look well in cabinets are, among others, otters, polecats, ferrets, weasels, foxes, rabbits, rats and mice. Perhaps you will find a dog most easy to practise upon. Well, the question naturally arises, where are you to procure a dead dog? This is easily enough answered as far as London is concerned, where, at the Home for Lost Dogs, York Road, Battersea, a large number of unfortunate strays are almost every week humanely destroyed. Mr. Pavitt, the head keeper, is exceedingly kind and obliging, and would not refuse to let you have a dead specimen. If you have the choice, get a somewhat small one ...

Taxidermy was one of a range of skills used by boys with an interest in natural history, a topic that was the subject of many B.O.P. articles and queries. And behind all of them was the Rev. J.G. Wood, a character as prolific and multifaceted as Dr Gordon Stables.

Chapter 9

==============================X==============================

'COMPANIONSHIP OF REPTILES'

The natural world of boys

We can but regret that any lad's friends should discourage his study of natural history on the ground that he is 'now growing to be a man, and should be thinking of something better;' and you have our sympathy in your uphill struggle. Stick to your hobby as long as you can, work at it thoroughly and conscientiously, and if you cannot convert your friends you may at least convert their children, and save them from becoming the victims of such stupidity.

Since the theme of manliness pervades the psyche of the B.O.P. writers, it's not surprising that the Editor would attempt to nip in the bud any suggestion that there was something wimpish about studying the flora and fauna of Victorian Britain. He was aided in this task by the Rev. J.G. Wood, a noted naturalist whose prolific pen and daring exploits make one wonder how he ever had time to take Matins in the church of St Thomas Martyr, Oxford, where he was curate and then priest for some time. But natural history eventually supplanted ministering to a parish and he made a career as a very successful writer and lecturer on natural history. His book *Common Objects of the Country* sold 100,000 copies *in its first week.*

Wood did a kind of double act with another writer, Arthur Stradling, whose writings dealt with far away places and exotic animals, while Wood was eager to show how much wild life there was around every boy if only he took the trouble to look. And a boy needed hardly any special equipment to 'naturalise' as Wood called it, as he explained in an article called *Out with a Jack-knife*.

> The Editor of this Magazine having asked me to show what could be done in Practical Natural History with no other apparatus than a common jack-knife, I have been out with such a weapon, and have had a capital time of it.... Only one blade is wanted. Many vendors try to dazzle their customers with complicated pieces of machinery which they are pleased to call universally useful knives.
>
> There are at least three blades, one large and two small. There is a corkscrew, which invariably doubles up across the fingers when used.
>
> There is an instrument for picking stones out of horses' hooves. It may be useful enough to those who ride or drive, but as we do not naturalise in a gig or on horseback, it is only in the way.
>
> There is a nutcracker, which might be used during the short time when the nuts are ripe, but is certainly not required for the rest of the year.
>
> There is a saw, which is quite superfluous; and there is a file, which is soon choked and rendered useless. There is a gimlet, a bradawl, and a rymer, and lastly come a pair of tweezers and a gun-picker. In practice, the saw, bradawl, gimlet, corkscrew, and rymer are soon broken, and the gun-picker and tweezers lost.
>
> Nothing is needed in a good, serviceable jack-knife but a single blade. No one wants to make pens when he is on a naturalising expedition, and if he did, the pens could not be used for want of ink.
>
> ... Always have your knife secured by a string and let the string be hung around the neck, but in such a way that if the

string be hitched in anything the loop will not tighten round the neck.

... Do not have the blade to open and close too easily, or it may shut up unexpectedly and cause a nasty wound. I once nearly lost the forefinger of my right-hand by such an accident.

I was working at the trunk of a tree, and leaning rather heavily on my knife, which shut with the edge over the finger, and had the full weight of my body on it. Thinking little of the cut, I wrapped my finger in a handkerchief, and went on with my work.

Presently the sun, which was shining brightly, became darkened; then the leaves and the grass turned black instead of green, and then it occurred to me that I was lying on the ground. I had fainted – for how long I cannot tell, but it must have been for some time, as I had fallen over an ant's nest, and the insects were swarming all over me.

More than thirty years have passed, but the scar is very conspicuous, just over the knuckles ...

In spite of Wood's strictures on the multi-bladed knife, the B.O.P. quite happily carried advertisements on the covers of its monthly numbers, for 'the J.P. Pocket Knife', with all the devices Wood condemned.

THE "J.P." POCKET KNIFE.

We have a glimpse of the working methods of this workaholic cleric in an article in the B.O.P.:

Often at his desk by five o'clock in the morning, much of his actual writing was done before breakfasting, as he sat surrounded by books and pamphlets, all bearing upon his favourite studies. Generally, a favourite cat lay curled up by his side; the floor would be littered with bones and skulls and horns, and other specimens innumerable; perhaps some exotic snails or half a dozen living scorpions would be in a cage at his elbow. And always outside his window, towards eight o'clock, would be a host of noisy, chattering, clamorous birds, all waiting impatiently for the breadcrumbs and porridge which he regularly prepared for them.

Immediately after breakfast came the day's correspondence, generally including queries upon natural history subjects from admirers in all parts of the habitable world. Then an hour or two would be devoted to the business connected with the well-known Sketch Lectures, which never satisfied himself and which he was always endeavouring to improve.

...After taking luncheon, and a short interval for necessary exercise or repose, Mr. Wood was accustomed to return to his desk and write almost continuously until nigh upon midnight. Always with two or three books in hand, besides magazine contributions innumerable MSS. seemed literally to flow from his pen ...

During his later years he was visited with threatenings of writer's cramp ... and he therefore adopted the use of a typewriter in the preparation of his MS. This accompanied him even by train, in the long and frequent journeys undertaken during his periodical lecture tours; and much speculation and interest were always excited in his fellow-passengers by the sight of the abstracted, fur-wrapped clergyman in the corner of the carriage, busily performing upon the keyboard of the strange machine.

Wood was a mainstay of the *Correspondence* pages, so much so that attempts were made to stem the tide of queries:

Rev. J.G. Wood hopes that his many young friends who address questions to him through the post will not feel hurt if he does not answer them through the same medium. The number of queries is simply appalling, and if he were to answer them through the post his whole time would be occupied in writing letters. He is glad to receive the queries, as they show a rapidly-increasing interest in Natural History, but, with a very few exceptions, the answers must be given in our Correspondence columns – that is, to such as are of general interest. We cannot afford the space for others.

– oOo –

We have sent your queries to the Rev. J.G. Wood, but he has so strong an objection to the caging of British wild birds, that he declines to answer any questions on the subject. Even if he did so, the answer would occupy several entire numbers of the BOY'S OWN PAPER, and we cannot spare this space.

– oOo –

We have sent your letter to the Rev. J.G. Wood, who says that he has often partaken of rat pie, and hopes to do so again. We never (knowingly) ate rats while we were living in Paris, but we did eat frogs occasionally.

Wood was useful to the B.O.P. in another way. As well as seeking factual information, 'our boys' would insist on sending dead specimens for identification, which meant that the B.O.P.'s postbox was sometimes clogged with tenuously wrapped boxes with unspeakable contents. It soon became the practice to send these on to Wood, encouraged by the Editor:

Feed it like any other squirrel. It is a small species. If it dies, you might send it at once to the Rev J.G.

Wood, who would doubtless be very glad to receive it.

In fact, as the *Correspondence* pages record, many packages were beyond redemption:

Your insect was smashed in the post; but we have identified the fragments as those of *Cetonia aurata*, the common rose-beetle. Next time you send us a specimen, put it in a box.

– oOo –

We did not receive the caterpillar, but, from your description, it had been attacked by the common ichneumon-fly (*Microgaster glomeratus*). Sixty or seventy of them are often found in one caterpillar. You ought to have enclosed your letter and specimens in the same parcel, as we cannot be expected to sort out and match a miscellaneous heap of letters, postcards, and parcels. If you saw our room after the delivery of the morning post, you would understand the necessity for this obvious precaution.

– oOo –

Let the care be yours to pack the parcel properly, and never send a packet through the post unless it is so done up as almost to defy damage. Rest assured that the postal authorities will never read more than the address. A box containing insects can of course be sent 'leagely,' as you call it; but 'with care' on the label is surplusage, as you can hardly expect it to come on in any special manner. It goes in the bag with the rest of the mail, and takes its chance, and the postmaster was correct in his statement, though unpardonably uncivil in the mode he made it.

– oOo –

Only half of your fly reached us, the packet having come to grief in the post. Why not pack more carefully? Of course we cannot identify the insect from the fragment received.

– oOo –

Your letter and its contents arrived in a most gruesome condition, mould prevailing to such a degree that much of the writing was quite illegible. The gall, too, was perfectly unrecognisable, and we cannot even hazard a guess as to its character. Do not pack anything in future until quite dry, or mould will be the inevitable result.

– o O o –

Like almost all those who send us birds' eggs to identify, you selected a box of the most fragile description, and packed it, moreover, without the least consideration for the energetic proceedings of the post-office officials. The natural result followed, and your eggs reached us in a condition of almost impalpable powder.

– o O o –

How do you expect us to name a bumble-bee which has first been pressed flat in a letter, and then pounded flatter still by some energetic postal authority? It is one of the red-hipped species, and that is all that we can say.

The other principal B.O.P. writer and naturalist, Dr Arthur Stradling, was somewhat scornful of boys who were content to have birds or mice as pets, oblivious to the wider world of more exotic animals whose interests he promoted in his articles.

Everybody knows all about guinea pigs and their habits, but how many boys, or grown-up people either, can tell the difference between a lizard and a newt? And which is the rarer feat, to teach a dog to sit up and beg, or to induce a frog to come at your call, and feed out of your hand?

Stradling had good credentials. 'From my cradle upwards,' he wrote, 'I have been accus-

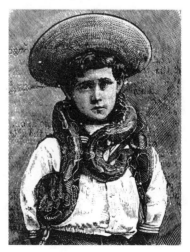

tomed to the companionship of reptiles ...' And to prove it, there is a picture of an angelic nine-year-old, festooned with a boa constrictor. To me, the young Arthur doesn't look as if he is enjoying the experience:

In later life, Stradling continued to show a particular fondness for snakes, which he sometimes called serpents:

> I have succeeded in bringing the eggs of foreign serpents to maturity in the tropics on the roof of a house, and in wet cotton-wool in the engine room of a steamer during a long voyage, though I have had many more failures than successes in that line. Once I carried about a number of coral snake's eggs in a flat tin case sewn inside the lining of my waistcoat for a considerable time, but no little scarlet and black creepers rewarded my patience.

Whenever, like Wood, he gave public lectures, he liked to terrify the audience by producing creatures from about his person. But this sometimes backfired:

> Last year, [Stradling wrote] I was giving a lecture on toads, illustrated with sixty or seventy specimens from all parts of the world, which were sent round amongst the audience in flat glass boxes for examination, and I lost one of these – a big African chap; but that is the only thing which I have ever had stolen from me on the lecture platform. It was rather too bad, on this occasion in particular, because, having had something to say about the edible frog and its possible acclimatisation in this country, I had procured at considerable trouble and expense, nearly two hundred of these edible frogs' legs from the Continent, and these – served hot on toast and in little patties – I distributed among those present at the conclusion of the lecture. A great joke it was, too! I did not expect they would eat them, but they did, every one, and took the bones home as curiosities. One

of the most celebrated animals ever received at the Zoological Gardens, a remarkable wolf, had been stolen before it reached there; and I was once just in time to drop a lasso over the shoulders of a man who was sneaking off with a tame leopard of mine.

Even when his snakes were dead, Stradling was not finished with them, and he used his experience to write an article called *What to do with a dead snake.*

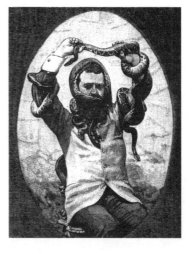

Between them, Stradling and Wood probably dealt with most of the B.O.P. nature queries. But Hutchison himself occasionally let slip that he, too, had a penchant for small furry animals:

Bats are far too wild and fond of their liberty to do well in confinement. We advise you to leave them alone. In our garden at Leytonstone we have quite a colony of them, and it is most interesting to watch them gnat-catching.

We know that was Hutchison because he had a house in Leytonstone, left when he died as a home for boys. But the other answers usually spoke in a generic B.O.P. voice:

Woodlice are crustaceans, and feed entirely upon decaying animal and vegetable substances. They are very fond of moisture, and during drought, or in dry spots, they are never to be seen. As to getting rid of them, our own experience is that one can't.

– oOo –

You ask a question which it would require hours to answer. An article on the subject appeared in our first volume. How can we possibly tell you on what to feed your caterpillars when you do not even say to what species they belong?

– oOo –

L.H. (Greenock) writes to us on what he thinks a very curious discovery. He says: 'A short time ago I had a duck's egg for breakfast, and when I had eaten it to the middle what was my astonishment (and I may say disgust) to see a small snail sticking half in the yolk and half in the white of the egg. It was quite dead, of course, having been boiled, but I suppose it would be dead before the egg was boiled. Now, sir, what I would like to know is this – How did the snail get into the egg? I may mention that the egg was perfectly fresh, except a slight blackness around the spot where the snail lay. If you can enlighten me with regard to this, I shall feel deeply grateful.' L.H. has not made any very wonderful discovery after all. It is not by any means an uncommon event to find foreign objects in eggs. The Rev. J.G. Wood, to whom we showed the letter, says he has seen three eggs one inside another. Lost rings have been found in eggs. In South Africa stones are almost always found in ostrich eggs.

– oOo –

THE CYANIDE BOTTLE – A.D.F. (Rochester) writes: 'I cannot think what your correspondent, S.J., has to find fault with, unless indeed his cyanide bottle has not been properly prepared. I find it most effective. The bottle may be carried in the pocket, opened to admit the moth, and closed again directly after it has entered. I have used it for several weeks, now that the season has begun, and find its power to have decreased little or nothing. If S.J. should be desirous of having his mixed in the same way as my own – which is cyanide of potassium and plaster of Paris, forming a solid mass – any chemist will do it for him for a very little.'

– oOo –

Very glad you like our paper, and speak so highly of the articles on 'Natural History for the Month.' Thanks for getting us new subscribers. You enjoy the reading of the BOY'S OWN yourself, and you seem to enjoy it far more when you get others to share your enjoyment. This certainly shows you have good in you. What ancient Grecian king or general was it who, whenever he had anything particularly nice for his dinner, was in the habit of sending a share of it to some of his favourite officers? We do not ask for information, but to test your knowledge. He was a good man. Spiders are preserved thus – you make an incision along the lower part with a very sharp knife, then remove the pulpy matter with a small forceps, then clear away the contents of the abdomen with a fine-pointed scissors till you can see the colour shining through. Afterwards blow out or extend the skin with a blow-pipe. You may have to repeat the blowing process several times until it sets. You may or may not set beetles with the wings showing. They look better without.

– oOo –

To relax insects, place a layer of damp sand in a jam-pot, or other vessel; pin the insects on the sand, and cover the jar. In about two days they will be perfectly relaxed. Zinc boxes are sold for this purpose. These boxes are fitted with cork instead of sand. The cork is wetted on the under surface, and the insects pinned on the other. Do not leave them too long, or they will mildew.

– oOo –

Snails often make a noise with the edge of their shells while crawling, especially upon glass.

– oOo –

Your butterfly is a specimen of the Small Tortoiseshell (*Vanessa urticae*). It is very common.

– oOo –

We should advise you to stuff your female Vapourer moth if you can, as otherwise she is sure to shrivel up and become almost unrecognisable. You can then either pin or set her out on card by means of gum, as you prefer. The larvae will eat almost any leaf, and are especially fond of pear, plum, and other fruit trees. Birch, too, is a favourite food.

– oOo –

Read our articles on Frogs and Toads in Vol. 1. The use of them? If it comes to that, what is the use of you? Does not the phrase, 'animals and their uses' strike you as savouring of presumption?

– o O o –

Observe all you can, but do not be dogmatic. No one can say that the cuckoo does not lay *in* and not *beside* the intended foster parents' nest as often as not. Birds can lift and carry their eggs, and many do; but what you assert is no proof that as regards the cuckoo this is always the case. We wish, however, that all our country readers were like you – observers, and sent us their experiences of what they saw and heard.

– o O o –

TONY THE 2nd – The Great Tit, Tony, still bears the evil reputation ascribed to him in old books; he still thinks that if he lays open the heads of other birds at all he may as well make a meal on the brains, which at best can be of little further use to the proprietor. But *does* he lay open the heads of other birds? That is an open question.

– o O o –

A book to tell you all the names and properties of every tree and plant in any part of the world would be, even in the smallest possible type on the thinnest possible paper, of such size and weight that you could not carry it about with you. There are books on the Amazons by Bates and Edwards that would give you the information you require.

– o O o –

It is not advisable to play tricks with any of the nightshades. They are all more or less poisonous. The most dangerous is the dwale – *Atropa belladonna* – the plant that gives the eye-wash. It is quite true that a vast number of British plants might be used for human food, but you should conduct your experiments very carefully, as you might make a mistake that would prove serious.

– o O o –

The value of collections of natural objects does not consist in what they will fetch, but in what they teach you.

– o O o –

We are sorry to say we are not able to identify your caterpillar. It is not an easy task. We are pretty good entomologists, but your description is not quite clear enough. He is not the right sort of caterpillar if he has sixteen legs. He is too original in his understanding.

– o O o –

A SNAIL-OPHOBIST – Suffer from snail-ophobia, do you? It is a new disease. And not liking to take away their little lives, you throw them into your neighbour's garden. Well, do you know that sounds mean, to say the least? And we do not blame the snails for crawling back either. Catch them and pop them into boiling water, or crush them with the heel of your boot, and give them to the fowls.

– o O o –

The 'Mr. Woods travelling about in a caravan full of insects, and that you may go and see them if he happens to be in the place where you are, but only unless you take in the B.O.P. regularly', is, we suppose, some remarkable version of Dr. Stables's tour in the Wanderer, for which see the last Summer Number.

– o O o –

Yes; by all means use the blackberry alone if you can obtain no other; but surely even in your district you can get the rowan also.

– o O o –

There is nothing remarkable in your 'snake' adventure. But go on studying natural history out of doors all the same.

– o O o –

Here is an answer to your question in the words of Lord Walsingham himself, who has been most successful in preserving caterpillars by the method referred to: 'A piece of watch-spring is heated at one end and twisted round the glass tube (blowpipe); the other end, which retains its spring and curve, presses on to the side of the tube, and, having a V-shaped mark in the extreme end, holds the skin while drying. . . There should be a bulge at the end of the tube, to assist in holding the skin on as it dries; it must, however, be very slight, or the skin will not come off again.'

– o O o –

The caterpillar reached us, but only as a corpse; and it was so shrivelled and dried that we cannot pretend to identify it. All we can say is, that it was one of the Geometers, or Loopers, which are often so exactly like pieces of twig that the keenest eye can scarcely detect them.

– oOo –

We cannot undertake to name parasites.

– oOo –

A STRANGE QUERY (F. Robinson) – Frank wants to know how to rear an oak tree from an acorn. Stick it in the ground, of course, and sit down and watch. In about two hundred years you may have a fine *tree*. If you only want to see the acorn sprout, stick the lower end in water in a glass vase.

– oOo –

A. B. O. E. wishes to know (1) how 'to get worms in bread as an object for the microscope,' and (2) how 'to burn the inside of an insect out to make it transparent.' We reply: 1. Let a little paste get sour, and keep it wet – there will soon be plenty of the 'eels,' as they are called. 2. Soak for several weeks in liquor potassae, squeeze out the interior, and mount in Canada balsam.

– oOo –

The beetle is *Creophilus maxillosus*. We thank you for the Hedgehog parasites, and will reply more fully to your question.

– oOo –

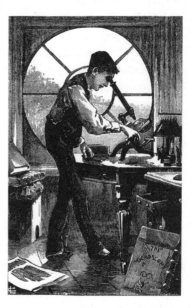

A. E. SANKEY (Gravesend) A correspondent, whose letter we have unfortunately mislaid, sent us some little time ago a large green caterpillar, which he had found in a potato-field. The larva is that of the Death's Head Hawk Moth (*Acherontia atropos*), which is remarkable for its power of squeaking when alarmed, in the pupal and perfect, as well as in the larval states. It is not usually a common insect, but the caterpillars seem to have been found in greater abundance than usual during the past season.

– oOo –

The autumn leaves you so kindly sent reached us quite safely, and are indeed very beautiful. We thank you heartily for thus remembering 'the Editor.'

– oOo –

INQIRER – Oh! Sure of an answer this time, as we dare not leave 'u' out. A great many plants of the natural order Umbelliferae will grow under trees. Unfortunately they are principally valuable for their foliage, and not for their flowers. Ivy will grow there, but nothing will do well that has a brilliant flower. There is too little sun and too much drip.

– oOo –

NEURASTHENIPPPONSKE-LESTERIZO – Your pseudonym is decidedly unique. The small flies enclosed are specimens of one of the ichneumon flies, *Microgaster glomeratus*, which preys upon the larvae of many destructive insects, thereby doing great service to the agriculturist.

– oOo –

We have here no room to 'explain the manners of the silkworms.'

A favourite pastime for boys was collecting and preserving specimens of wildlife. But before a creature could become a specimen you had to kill it. How to cause death and what to do with a corpse was a constant motif in the *Correspondence* columns.

Pinch the butterfly sharply at the junction of the legs, and it will instantly die. If a butterfly in the net is thus killed at once, it will not be damaged. Forceps are better than fingers for this purpose.

– oOo –

Three or four minutes ought to be sufficient for killing a butterfly in the cyanide bottle. You had better pinch the thorax smartly on taking it out, to make matters certain. Moths must be left in for a longer time.

– o O o –

Drop the shell into boiling water, and the animal will come out like a periwinkle. Death is instantaneous.

– o O o –

The most satisfactory way of obtaining the skeleton of a small animal is to put the dead body into soft water and let it macerate.

– o O o –

We are afraid that we cannot suggest an improvement on the barbarism to which you allude. You can try stabbing with a steel pen dipped in strong oxalic acid, if you like, and if you can induce your butterfly to lie quietly in the net while you get out the bottle and make your preparations. If he is a fluffy butterfly, however, most of the acid will be brushed off the pen before it enters the body. Read articles on 'Killing Insects' in Nos. 27 and 28, and on 'Treacling' in Nos. 9 and 10. English collectors use

rounded setting-boards, and leave the insects low upon the pins. Continental entomologists use flat boards, and run the pin through the body almost as far as the head.

– o O o –

Break the fishes' necks by bending the head right back on the spine.

– o O o –

Depends whereabouts the wasps' nests are. Blow up with gunpowder if you can, or insert a lighted squib, in the composition of which sulphur predominates. But before this note can appear your troubles will probably be over.

– o O o –

To kill the larger beetles, dash them into <u>boiling</u> water when they will die instantaneously ...

– o O o –

You can hardly be a friend to snakes if you want to kill them. In our adventures with snakes, which have been many and varied and in all parts of the world, we have always thought more of preserving our own skin than the snake's. But if we were to catch a viper with long forceps, as the man in the

New Forest does, we should pop him into a bottle of gin.

– o O o –

Skin the mouse, and put it close to an ant's nest. You will soon have a clean skeleton.

– o O o –

Hang the dead fish in water and let the tadpoles eat it. You will soon get it skeletonised, but some of the parts may get taken away.

– o O o –

To whiten your skeleton and clean away the fatty emanations and disagreeable odour, rest the bones upon strips of zinc placed about an inch above the bottom of a glass jar, and fill it up with spirits of turpentine. The turpentine acts as an oxydising agent, and the product of the combustion is an acid liquor, which sinks to the bottom.

– o O o –

The only satisfactory way of procuring a skeleton is by maceration, which is odoriferous but sure. The other method is all very well, but in the first place you have to find the hill, and in the second you have to provide against the body being removed by some other agency.

– o O o –

To skeletonise any animal the simplest plan is first to denude it of all flesh and soft stuff, then put the bones down by an ants' nest. Protect from dogs or cats, however.

– o O o –

Almost the only satisfactory way of skeletonising birds, etc., is to leave them in soft water, and let them rot. It is a long process, and an odoriferous one, but it is effective. Insects have no bones. 2. To paint on glass mix your colours with varnish.

– o O o –

To preserve squirrel skins, scrape them, clear them of every fragment of fat, and rub them over with a soap made of a pound of yellow soap, and an ounce each of lime, camphor, arsenic, and alum. Another way is to nail the skins on a board and cover them with wood ashes for a fortnight, renewing the ashes every three days.

– o O o –

Thanks for your letter and your kind wishes. But before this can

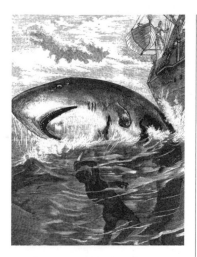

reach you your interesting young shark, who must have been a very lively youth indeed, will be too far gone to set up. Dr. Gordon Stables, R.N., has written a series for this paper on Taxidermy, and will give full instructions how to stuff and set up fishes, as well as birds and beasts.

– oOo –

DICK HARDEN – Your best plan will be to write to any of the London taxidermists, and specify the kind of birds'-eyes which you require. You will find their names in the Post Office Directory, under the heading of 'Naturalists.'

It's difficult to suppress a degree of admiration for the boys who took the B.O.P. articles at their word and set to work to follow detailed instructions, whether for building a dinner gong or an outboard engine, or stuffing a dead pet. Even when recommending the killing of birds for stuffing, the B.O.P.'s writers sounded a humane note:

> The wholesale destruction, for the sheer love of taking life, which goes on at all seasons round our seacoasts, is simply appalling. It is trusted that these hints on bird-stuffing may not stimulate it, but rather, by leading boys to take an interest in the marvellous structure of bird life, to venerate and spare it, shooting only here and there a solitary specimen for preservation ...

The first of many articles on taxidermy, in the second volume, was called *Birds and Beasts and How to Stuff Them,* and every year or two the B.O.P. returned, presumably by popular demand, to the topic.

> As in all probability tiger and buffalo skins will not come in the way of the readers of these lines,' one article said, 'it is rather such "small deer" as the denizens of our English woods they will be anxious to preserve, to wit, foxes' heads, cats, otters, stoats, weasels, moles, or water-rats. But the following hints apply equally to a tiger-skin or a squirrel's.
>
> Let us begin by imagining the keeper has brought in a fine large poaching cat. Take the beast to an outhouse, and in the shade lay it on its back, and with a butcher's, or indeed any sharp knife, make a long, straight, but not too deep cut, from the centre of the lower jaw to the end of the tail. Then cut down the legs on the underneath side till the cut down the centre of the body is reached. Now separate the skin from the body ...

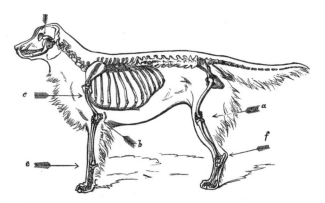

Articles on taxidermy read every bit as gruesomely as tales of big game hunting or cannibalism:

> Mid-winter or mid-summer is the best time to shoot birds for stuffing, as when they have been recently sitting, or moulting, their feathers are apt to be worn or only half formed. Be

careful to use only small shot and small charges, at short distances, for small birds, or the skin will be irretrievably damaged. Increase the charge in proportion to the size of the bird, but it should never be a very heavy one. A friend once brought me to stuff a tame parrot of his which had flown away. Thinking to injure the skin the less, he had shot it with a charge of peas, but with the result of crushing it almost to a jelly, tearing the skin so it was useless.

The Head. – If the head is very much larger than the neck, cut the throat lengthways to remove the head. It is immaterial whether the eyes are taken out before the head is skinned or after. The gouge should go well to the back of the eye and separate the ligament which holds it to the socket. Should the gouge go into the eye, it will let out the moisture, which often damages the skin. Some people crush the skull slightly to make it come out of the skin easily, but this I do not advise. Remove the brains by taking out a piece of the skull at the back as you cut off the neck. Pull the eyes out of their cavity and fill up their place with wool soaked in arsenical soap. Anoint the skin of the head and the neck well with arsenical soap, and place in the neck a piece of stick red with wool, the end of which put into the hole made in the skull for extracting the brains ...

In 1889, the B.O.P. had to publish a sad letter from a correspondent. It began, 'The death of the Rev J.G. Wood is an irreparable loss to the boys of England, and especially to the readers of the B.O.P. ...'

The writer added the following paragraph:

It grieves me very much to see that his wife and family are left in a state of comparative destitution. I am sure thousands of your readers will be glad of an opportunity of showing their appreciation of Mr. Wood's unwearied labours on their behalf by subscribing their sixpences to a B.O.P. fund for assisting his widow and orphans ...

In spite of his lecture tours and his best-selling books, Wood had apparently died leaving his family in poverty. But the B.O.P. and its readers were good at rallying round when need arose – they had raised money for a Boy's Own lifeboat and a boys' hostel during its first few years – and so a fund was soon set up to relieve the Wood family's poverty. History doesn't show who was now the addressee of choice for the stream of broken butterflies and disintegrating starlings that B.O.P. readers continued to send.

In the *Answers to Correspondents* columns, there was no predicting which queries would be given short shrift and which would have the indulgence of a long and detailed answer. Some of the longest answers consisted of recipes, sometimes for foods or drinks, but sometimes for purposes that were much less clear. With the following answers, where the purpose is unclear from the recipe itself, it is given in a list at the end.

1. Boil three-quarters of a pound of lump sugar in a quarter of a pint of water, pour it while boiling hot on to six eggs, the whites and yolks whisked for two minutes. Beat up the eggs and sugar till they become a thick batter. Mix in lightly and quickly ten ounces of good white flour, put into buttered tins, and bake in a moderate oven. The flavouring should be added while the eggs are being whisked.

2. Take 1½lb lump sugar and 1oz. citric acid (lump), and dissolve in one quart boiling water. When cold, add one dessert-spoonful of essence of lemon. Bottle and keep well corked. One tablespoonful added to a tumbler of water will make excellent lemonade.

3. Put some concentrated solution of zinc chloride into a porcelain or copper vessel, dilute it with not more than two volumes of water, and boil. Should there be a precipitate dissolve it with a few drops of hydrochloric acid. Take as much powdered zinc on the point of a knife as it will hold, and throw it into the mixture, and the vessel will then receive an internal coating of zinc. Now add either chloride or sulphate of nickel until the water is distinctly green, and then put in the articles you wish to plate, having first well cleaned them, and boil them up with some zinc fragments for a quarter of an hour. Wash them well with cold water, and clean with chalk. If the covering of nickel is not thick enough, go through the process again.

4. The best sort of whitewash we know is that used at the President's residence at Washington, the so-called White House. It is made as follows: Half a bushel of good unslaked lime is slaked with boiling water, and covered during the process to keep in the steam. The liquor is carefully strained and mixed with a peck of salt which has been dissolved in warm water; three pounds of good rice are then ground to a thin paste and stirred in while boiling hot, and there are also added half a pound of powdered whiting and a pound of glue made in the usual way, and added when hot and clear. Five gallons of hot water are then stirred into the mixture, which is then kept for a few days in a covered cask to settle. It is put on quite hot and one pint will cover a square yard of ordinary brickwork.

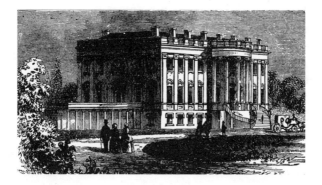

5. Ordinary whitewash is merely whiting and size, and this, if properly made and laid on a clean surface, will not wash off. A good whitewash is made by mixing six balls of whiting with two pounds of size and one ounce of blue-black. Melt the size in a kettle, and pour it on to the whiting when hot. The American lighthouses are said to have the finest whitewash in the world. [*So, six years after recipe 4, the White House has been displaced in the whitewash stakes by American lighthouses.*]

6. First melt the copper in a plumbago crucible, and immerse the whole of the zinc, which must be dry and cool, when the copper is only just fluid. Drop a piece of borax as big as a walnut into the pot, and cover the surface of the hot metal with a layer of fine charcoal, which you must keep renewing as it burns.

7. Let the broken material, bricks, pebbles, or what not, you use with your cement, be broken into about two-inch cakes. Use Portland cement costing about 2s. 9d. per bushel. Mix your concrete on a board, so as to keep it clear from dirt. Water gradually, and only on the heap you are working at, and mix thoroughly. A good mixture for your purposes would be five parts of gravel and sand to one part of fresh-burned stone lime.

8. Boil a pound of log-wood in four quarts of water, and then add a double-handful of walnut-shells. Then boil it up again, take out the shells, and add a pint of vinegar. Put it on hot. The cheapest way is to buy a sixpenny bottle of stain. Gold-size thickened with vegetable-black will give you a black paint that might do.

9. Make some paper putty by steeping the flimsiest of newspapers in a smooth paste of a pound of wheat flour, a tablespoonful of ground alum, and three quarts of water, and plug up all the holes and cracks. Then give the floor a coat of thin paste, and lay down a coat of stout manila or hardware paper. Wait till it is dry, and add another coat of coarse paper. When that is dry give it a good even coat of thin paste, and put down your wallpaper; a good geometrical pattern is the best - *not* the same as that on the walls of your room. Let your floor get perfectly dry, and then give it three separate coats of size made by dissolving a pound of white glue in a gallon of hot water. When that is dry give it a coat

of hard oil-finish varnish. This floor can be washed and cleaned like a wooden one, and if the paste has been put on properly it will wear for years.

10. The powder for green luminous paint is made by heating thio-sulphate of strontium for a quarter of an hour over a good Bunsen flame, and then for five minutes over a blast-lamp; that for blue luminous paint is made by heating equal parts of carbonate of strontium and milk-of-sulphur gently for five minutes, then strongly for twenty-five minutes over a Bunsen burner, and then finally for five minutes over a blast-lamp. You must, of course, expose the objects coated with these paints to the daylight. [*And don't be surprised if you develop cancer later in life.*]

11. To stain leather blue, boil elderberries, and soak the leather in them. Then boil the berries with alum-water, and again soak the leather in the liquid. To dye it green, boil sap-green in alum-water, and soak it well. To dye it yellow, smear it over with aloes and linseed-oil. To dye it sky-blue, soak it in a warm solution of indigo, which has been made by steeping the indigo in water for twelve hours and then boiling it. Or try the aniline dyes.

12. Dissolve half an ounce of cyanide of potassium in a wine-glass of water, and immerse the steel in the mixture until all the dirt and rust is cleaned off it. Then make a paste of Castile soap, cyanide of potassium, whiting, and water, and brush the article well over with it. To keep steel from rusting coat it with boiled linseed oil and let it dry on; or dissolve an ounce of camphor in two pounds of hog's lard, and after skimming it stir in as much blacklead as will make it look like iron. Rub the articles over with this stuff, and leave them for twenty-four hours before you clean them down with a linen cloth. Machinery sent abroad is coated with this blackleading. [*If father should come home and attempt to drink from the wineglass, advise him against it.*]

13. Try a mixture of twenty pounds of river sand, two pounds of litharge, and a pound of quicklime mixed up into a paste with raw linseed oil.

14. Take a Swede turnip (which can be kept through the whole year by burying it in sand in a cool place), grate it fine, immerse some crumb of white bread in water, squeeze it dry, add a handful of barley-meal, and mix all together in a pestle and mortar. Five parts rape and one part canary is the best seed food for chaffinches. Do not forget that rape-oil is castor-oil, and that the seeds have a similar tendency to be laxative, so that a little bruised rice is good occasionally.

15. Boil three ounces of powdered ginger and five pounds of loaf-sugar in three gallons of water for an hour, and let the solution cool. Add to it, then, the juice and peel of five lemons; then put in a quarter of a teacupful of yeast spread on a slice of toasted bread. Cover the pan with a thick cloth, and do not touch it for three days. Then strain the liquor through a cloth, and bottle it. In a week you will find it ready for drinking. If you like the taste of ginger to be very strong, use five ounces instead of three. Follow these directions carefully; do not attempt to improve on them, and your ginger-beer will have only one fault - there will not be enough of it.

16. Wet a piece of rag with antimony chloride, dip it into olive-oil, and rub the barrel. In forty-eight hours it will be covered with a coat of rust, which you can remove with a scratch-brush, and then finish the barrel with a coat of oil.

17. Take two pounds of common salt, a quarter of a pound of bay salt, four pounds of saltpetre, two ounces of sal prunella, and two pennyworth of cochineal, which mix and pound together. Then get a peck of sprats. Put a layer of sprats, unwiped and unwashed just as received, into a stone jar, and on them put a layer of mixture; then add a layer of sprats, then one of mixture. When the jar is full press the contents well together, and cork it up for six months, when the 'anchovies' will be quite 'the finest Gorgona'.

18. Ground white sugar, essence of lemon, tartaric acid, and carbonate of soda. Pour forty drops of the lemon on half a pound of the sugar and mix them well together, and then add to the mixture a pound each of the soda and acid. It should be very well mixed.

19. For blue fire take thirty parts each of sulphur, sulphate of potash, and ammonia sulphate of copper, fifty-four parts of nitre, and fifty-six parts of chlorate of potash. Or, mix ten parts of nitre with four parts of sulphur and two parts of metallic antimony. For red fire mix seventeen parts of chlorate of potash, twenty-three parts of charcoal, ninety parts of sulphur, and 270 parts of nitrate of strontium. For green fire mix seventy-seven parts of nitrate of barytes, eight parts of chlorate of potash, three parts of charcoal, and thirteen parts of sulphur. But pray be careful.

20. Oil a square or round tin with low edges - a canister-lid is as good as anything. Split some almonds, and put them in rows on the bottom, with the split side downwards, until the surface is covered. Then boil some raw sugar to 'crack,' and pour it into the tin till it covers the almonds. 'Crack' is a technical term much used in confectionery, and is descriptive of a certain stage in boiling sugar. Get a jug of clean cold water and a round stick. Dip the stick in the water, then in the boiling sugar, then in the water again. If the sugar is slipped off the stick, and breaks short and crisp with a slight noise, it is boiled to 'crack;' if it can be rolled into a ball between the finger and thumb in the water, it is

at 'ball,' and is not done enough. The different stages are 'feather,' 'candy,' 'ball,' 'crack,' and 'caramel.' When you boil sugar, put the lid half on the pan as soon as the boiling begins.

21. Mix together in a basin three pounds of flour, half a pound of coarse brown sugar, two ounces of ground ginger, and an ounce of ground allspice; warm half a pound of butter, and add it, with two pounds of treacle, to the mixture in the basin. Take the chill off half a pint of milk in which you have dissolved two table-spoonfuls of carbonate of soda, whisk up half a dozen eggs, and then mix the milk, the eggs, and the contents of the basin into a smooth dough. Butter a tin, pour in the mixture, and bake it till it is done, which will be in an hour or two.

22. 'Is it possible to cook sardines?' Why not look in a cookery-book, and see for yourself? Here is one way we used to try with success. We took one of the large boxes holding a dozen, opened it, and warmed it so as to make the oil quite liquid, and then we carefully fished out the sardines. Then we took all the skins off the fish, and laid the fish out on a plate over the fire, or in the oven to get hot. Then we poured all the oil out of the tin into a little saucepan and boiled it, and as it boiled, stirred in a table-spoon of flour, and then we gradually added a very little water. The mixture thickened up to the consistency of cream, and we added to it a teaspoonful of Worcester or some other sauce, and some salt, and the least pinch of cayenne. Then we beat up together the yolk of an egg, a teaspoonful of French mustard, and a teaspoonful of vinegar, and then we poured the hot sauce into this, and then the whole mixture into the hot sardines. The sardines treated in this way were excellent, but we left other people to clean the saucepan, etc., after us!

23. Get a few pennyworths of litharge from a chemist's, add to it an equal quantity of fine white dry sand, and an equal quantity

of plaster-of-Paris, and mix with it a third of its quantity of powdered resin. Take some boiled linseed oil, with a little dryers in it, and make your powder into a paste. Let it stand for four hours, and then use.

24. Salt the water; when boiling sprinkle in slowly the oatmeal (not too fine ground), stirring all the time until thick; then, after a minute or two; pour out into basins and cover with cold new milk; and after letting stand a little time to cool it is ready for eating; or, cover a saucer with cheese crumbs, pour in the porridge, and let it cool, and then turn it out on to a plate.

25. Two ounces of clear gum arabic, an ounce and a half of fine starch, and half an ounce of white sugar. Pulverise the gum and dissolve it in as much water as would be just sufficient for the starch, and then add the starch to the solution. Then cork the mixture in a vessel suspended in boiling water until the starch becomes clear and the cement is as thick as tar. Add to it a little oil of cloves, or sassafras, and it will keep for months.

26. Put a sponge cake into a deep china or glass dish; pour round it some white wine, and then strew sifted sugar over it, and pour in the dish a rich thick custard, according to your fancy.

27. Take one ounce of lemon juice, a quarter of a drachm of powdered borax, and half a drachm of sugar; mix and let them stand a few days in a glass bottle till the liquor is fit for use; then rub it on the hands and face occasionally.

28. Cement a thin piece of indiarubber over it. Get sixpenny-worth of benzine (free from grease) from a druggist, and add to it a tenth of its volume of indiarubber cut into fine shreds. In a day or two the indiarubber will be all melted, and you will have a cement which will unite almost anything, not only in the indiarubber way, but in the leather way as well.

Answers:

1. Sponge cake

6. For smelting brass

7. 'Two bushels of concrete will cover two and a quarter yards, one inch deep. From this you can calculate the quantity required for your court.'

8. To ebonise a very large surface

9. How to wallpaper your floor

13. To mend a window sill

14. 'A genuine German paste for chaffinches and small birds generally'

16. To brown a gun-barrel

17. 'Anchovies come from the Mediterranean – in theory. In practice "we make them ourselves".'

18. Sherbet

19. *Your guess is a good as mine*

20. 'We have given several ways of making toffee, butter-scotch, and hardbake. Refer to back numbers. Here is another way that may suit you if you omit the almonds.'

23. This is the mixture used to cement the glass to the frames in the fish-house at the Zoological Gardens

24. Porridge-making in Cumberland and Westmoreland

25. A substance called Winchell's Paste which is said to stick anything, even glazed surfaces

26. To make a 'tippling cake'

27. To disperse freckles

=X=

'ALL INTERFERENCE IS RUINOUS...'

Keeping up appearances

> Boys of about sixteen often ask us strange questions about their
> feelings and sensations [wrote Gordon Stables] and strange
> things that happen to them about this time. These are natural,
> and *all* interference is ruinous. Be warned!

Among the strange things that happened to boys at that time were
the appearance or non-appearance of facial hair. Those who
didn't have it wanted it; those who had it wanted more – or less –
of it; and those who had the right amount weren't sure if it was in
the right places.

It's easy to forget how important beards and moustaches were
in late Victorian times, only because they were far more prevalent
than they are today. Portraits of popular sportsmen showed them
regularly sporting facefuls of hair that would have made any
bare-faced boy feel inferior.

Bearing in mind the wide age range at which puberty starts, it
only required the presence of one or two hairily-precocious boys
in the class to set the rest wondering if they were freaks of nature
and doomed to perpetual smoothness.

A B.O.P. poem, called *A Shaver's Experience*, began:

> Oh, what were my feelings one morning when I
> Left my soft downy couch with a long weary sigh,
> And as often before raised my hand to my chin,

And found a strange substance had grown on the skin!
With a wild shriek of joy I rushed to the glass,
In hopes what I longed for had now come to pass.
I was rather in doubt, for it struck me just then
That last night, in our fight with 'dormitory ten,'
When I hit that young Brown a crack on the head
That sent him back howling in anger to bed,
I had heard my old pillow go off with a squeak.
Just suppose that this substance was caused by a leak
In my pillow – that feathers it was that had stuck on my chin!
I seized the cracked glass, and in terror looked in;
No, it was not feathers, there wasn't a doubt
Of 'the soft down of manhood' beginning to sprout!
I shrieked, and I danced, and I stood on my head,
I believe I turned head over heels on my bed ...

'How to shave' was one of a number of queries about general hairiness:

We can*not* promise a series of articles on 'Shaving.' The subject is one of wide interest, we admit, but it is scarcely suitable for our columns! Surely you can restrain your impatience to divest yourself of the 'incipient down' until you meet with some one who can explain to you the not very occult mysteries of razor and lather-brush!

– oOo –

The 'best thing for a boy to do who is nervous of the first operation of shaving' is either to leave the operation alone, or to procure a convex mirror. In it, his countenance will assume such an enlarged and gleeful expression that all his fears will evaporate and the dreadful ordeal will be got through with ease!

– oOo –

Like learned Fusbos, we cannot advise. Perhaps our readers may suggest something. 'I am very much bothered with my hair. It is so stubborn and thick that I cannot part it, and grows very low over my forehead. I have tried a good many dressings for the hair, but they have not had the desired effect,' whatever that may be!

– oOo –

Leave your grey hairs alone. Such cases are not common, but there is no reason why a boy should be ashamed of grey hairs any more than an old man is. As you get out in the world you will find it do you no harm to be thought a little older than you are, particularly if you start in a business on your own account.

– oOo –

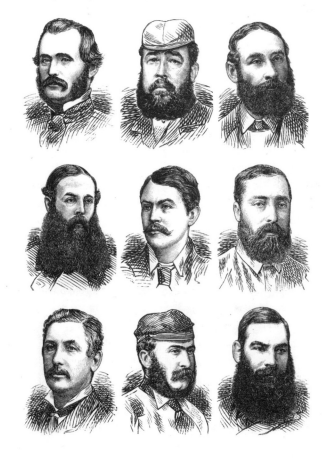

'Is it possible to transplant a hair from your head to your arm, so that it will grow there? When I say transplant, I mean to make a little hole in your arm with a needle, to pull a hair from your head, and to put the root into the hole.' We have never heard of this being done, but you could easily experiment for yourself. A single specimen would hardly be a fair test, so perhaps it would be as well to prod yourself over with two or three dozen needle-holes!

– o O o –

Ordinary perfumed olive oil. But nothing will make strong, stubby hair lie in the right direction.

– o O o –

1. 'Will forcing the growth of a moustache injure the roots of the hair?' Well, in the case of persons of weak mental development the roots of the hair are not at a very great distance from the moustache, and injury might arise, so that we think you had better be cautious! 2. Alexander Selkirk was the marooned sailor whose story was the foundation of that of 'Robinson Crusoe.' His hair grew naturally. The luxuriance you notice in the story-books was not the result of any forcing. Is it not possible that you have mistaken the hairy cap for a growth on his head? Some of the Crusoe illustrations are quite obscure enough to mislead you!

– o O o –

This young lady wants to know how to get rid of a few hairs growing on the face, also how many volcanoes there are in the world! Pull the hairs, if few, out with the tweezers. As to the volcanoes, we should not like to hazard even a guess.

But it was the moustache that was the source of greatest worry. Faced with a regular torrent of queries about missing or unbalanced moustaches, the Editor's usual recourse was to humour, coupled sometimes with reassurance.

We really do not think it desirable to promote the growth of whiskers amongst our readers. You must wait for your whiskers. If they come, well and good; if they do not, you will be saved a great deal of trouble and waste of valuable time. Men are never satisfied. Those who have no whiskers seem to be miserable till they get them, and those that have them would in many cases be only too glad to get rid of them.

– o O o –

Are you so very anxious to have moustachios? If nature does not endow you with them, we can recommend you no specific: nor can we tell you how to grow tall!

– o O o –

The simplest way of promoting the growth of whiskers is to grow older at the rate of seven days a week. Wash your face frequently with soap and water, and wait till the crop appears.

– o O o –

We are rejoiced to hear that you weigh ten stone two pounds, and hope by this time that 'the signs of a moustachio,' so ardently desired by you, have duly appeared. There is no occasion for alarm even if the merest shadow of an eyebrow has not yet risen into view. Live on in hope.

– o O o –

A CONSTANT READER (not the only one by any means, but a peculiar one) desires 'a good prescription for growing a whisker.' Only one, O Constant Reader? Are you like unto Good in King Solomon's Mines? Rub your bare cheek with Vaseline, and let the sun shine on it all you can!

– o O o –

There seems to be quite a run on them this week. First 'A Moustachios Admirer' tells us, 'I am the eldest of five, and all my other brothers are growing a moustachios but me; could you please give me an answer how to make mine grow?' Why not apply to your 'other brothers,' O A.M.A.? Then F.C.L. 'wishes to know what is the best way to get a moustache? Are the advertisements as to Mrs. Allen's hair restorer of any use?' Yes, of great use - for the sale of the article. Then '*Causa sine qua non*' says, 'My apology for a moustache will only grow at the corner, and a friend told me that hot beverages like tea, etc., scalded the ends off and prevented them growing!' Clearly there is nothing like labouring and waiting!

– o O o –

Keep your lip close-shaven for a month or two, and use vaseline as if it were cold cream. Any preparation of petroleum will make the hair grow.

– o O o –

J. SMITH wishes to know 'the best way to force whiskers, etc.'; he has 'rubbed his face with vaseline,' but finds it 'no good whatever.' He is 'now over 20,' and his object in life is 'to grow a moustache' as a sort of municipal ornament for Newcastle-on-Tyne. Will the Kyrle Society, for the beautification of our cities, kindly oblige?

– o O o –

It must be annoying! 'My hair (on my head) is brown, and moustache quite a ginger or carrots.' Some vegetable preparation might help you? But it is best never to say dye. Why have a moustache, if you cannot get one of a colour to suit?

– o O o –

Wash the hair once a week, using a very mild soap. Moustache 'forcers' are of no good, except to the pockets of the quacks who recommend them.

– o O o –

IGNORAMUS – You cannot stop hair growing on your face. If you are too young to have a moustache you must keep your lips shaved, that is all; and you can keep on shaving for the rest of your life or let your moustache grow when you are older. The shaving will do no harm in either case.

– o O o –

IGNORAMUS (another of them, and on the very opposite tack. Why is it that when men have moustaches they want to get rid of them, and when they have none they want to 'cultivate' them?) – 'Does hair come from seed?' Well, not exactly! 'If so, can I get some from the doctor's shop?' Can you doubt it, O, Ignoramus – if that be the vocative – why not try the experiment, visit the nearest chemist and ask him for threepennyworth of whisker-seed?

– o O o –

We regret the delay in informing you how 'to grow a long silken moustache'; but we have written to a person who keeps Maltese terriers, as being likely to know, and when we receive his reply we will print it – if we have room.

– o O o –

It may be due to the presence of a bacillus attacking it. We should advise you to consult a doctor. This may be reason of the baldness also, especially if the hair got brittle or clubbed or curled up. Shaving the moustache would not in that case effect a cure. But the case is one for personal consultation.

– oOo –

VERY ANXIOUS – And pardonably so! 'I am fifteen years of age, and my moustachious are coming too fast; please insert in the Correspondence of the B.O.P. how to stop them, at least until I am 18.' Can any of our readers oblige this anxious youth whose hair is too apparent? He wants no dangerous nostrum which would keep his beard back until the pressure becomes so great on the eve of his eighteenth birthday that in the silence of the night the hair has to burst forth with a loud explosion like an aloe on the bloom and cover his face with a three years' growth, but some nice soft liniment that will prevent the undue growth of hair at the expense of intellect.

– oOo –

PIMPLED FACE – We regret that we are unprovided with the address of a respectable 'whisker-stopper,' and are quite unable to inform you how it is that 'ministers have their faces so smooth and clean.' As far as cleanliness is concerned we of course agree with you, but as to smoothness – well, you should not generalise too rashly. Judging from your pseudonym, we would timidly suggest as an alternative that you 'stop' your pimples and grow your whiskers. This would be 'the best thing for a pimpled face.'

Pimples, blackheads and other skin complaints were also the bane of boys' lives at their most self-conscious time. Many boys seem to have got the idea that such blemishes were caused by small creatures inhabiting their faces:

The marks on the face are specks, not worms. The lotion you mention is five grains of bichloride of mercury, an ounce of honey-water, and seven ounces of bitter almonds. It is poisonous, and we know nothing of its efficacy. You have to squeeze out your specks twice a day, and immediately apply the lotion. You had far better consult a doctor; if you case is not serious enough for that, leave your face alone.

– oOo –

The best way probably to get rid of 'the grubs' from the face would be to squeeze them out. The process may be painful, but it is sure.

– oOo –

Blackheads in face are often caused by poverty of blood and want of free circulation in vessels of face. They are not worms, as you think, but accumulations of sebaceous matter. Squeeze out, and apply twice a day a lotion of one grain of corrosive sublimate (poison) to an ounce of eau-de-cologne. Take a bark tonic, and keep system open by drinking cream-of-tartar water.

– oOo –

The ticks in the face are caused by debility of the skin. Use plenty of soap and a rough towel. Squeeze them out.

– oOo –

We may give more 'Boy's Troubles' soon. You can wait. Pimples do not kill.

– oOo –

It is difficult to give you a good remedy for pimples. A little diluted ointment of the nitrate of mercury is probably the best application, but the blood should be kept pure by good wholesome food and good wholesome exercise in the open air.

– oOo –

'SCURVY' ON THE FACE – You mean scurf not scurvy. It is a symptom of bad health. Attend to digestion and rules of health. Use a little benzoated oxide of zinc every night.

Tattoos, either amateur ones or professionally administered, were a source both of adornment and anxiety. The B.O.P. reported an extreme example of the practice:

A tramp was lately apprehended by the Leicester police, he having been found 'climbing a lamp-post to get a drink.' He was, when searched, found to be tattooed from his shoulders to his feet, the police description of his marks being: 'Letter D and ship on breast, together with a house, pigeons, anchor and chain, haystack, fishes and trees, a man driving a sheep, a pig, the Union Jack, the Prince of Wales's feathers, an anchor, two inscriptions, "Love me and leave me not" (Shakespeare), and a gravestone to "The memory of all I love," a Highland girl dancing, a Highland soldier and another soldier wearing a red coat, crossflags and a bayonet, drum and sticks, a pile of shot, W.F., a gun, another gun and crossed flags, crossed pipes, and a jug and glass; on the right arm an ensign, sailors, a ship, a cross and a large fish, a sailor with crossed flags, and "CHARLOTTE" in capital letters; on the left arm a policeman taking a man into custody, and Faith, Hope and Charity; on the left leg a man; on the right leg a woman and a flag.' Could any folly well exceed this?

Well, on a smaller scale, there was the folly of boys who acquired tattoos unthinkingly without realising that they might not want them in perpetuity:

Having tattooed your hand with Indian ink you must leave the marks there for the rest of your life. You could do a certain amount of good by warning your schoolfellows against indulging in such a foolish practice, and instancing yourself as an example. Prevention is better than cure.

– oOo –

In a few instances tattoo marks have been got rid of by criminals in Australia and elsewhere as a means of concealing their identity, but it is a very uncertain process, a painful one, and generally leaves a worse disfiguration than at first. As the real reason why tattooing is practised by sailors is that, if drowned, their corpses may be identified, the 'best pattern' you could select would be perhaps your name and address in full, and any particulars as to age and pedigree that you may think would prove interesting!

– oOo –

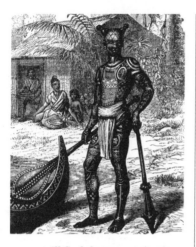

... you will find that your tattooings will take a lot of sucking before they disappear.

– oOo –

You had much better leave yourself alone. We are in receipt of dozens of letters from boys who have been foolish enough to tattoo themselves, asking us how to remove the marks.

– oOo –

Tattoo marks, if properly done, are indelible. We have seen them on the arms of old sailors, done when they were lads. Destruction of the skin by scalding is the only way of getting rid of them, but there would be risk of causing erysipelas, which is often fatal.

This was good advice. Erysipelas killed Princess Amelia, daughter of George III, although there is no evidence that this was in the course of trying to remove her tattoos.

Then, as now, boys were often unhappy about their general appearance – eyes, noses, ears and the rest of their genetic endowment. Although there was little that could be done to change these, 'our boys' lived in hope and pestered the Editor for solutions:

EYEBROWS MEETING (An Afflicted Reader) – We are inclined to say 'Afflicted Fiddlesticks.' Why should you worry over this? Thank Heaven you have health; and be a man.

– oOo –

EYEBROWS MEETING – Nothing to be done.

– oOo –

There are many advertised specifics for 'scant eyelashes' but we cannot undertake to recommend them. Some few persons believe in clipping, and most others in letting nature alone.

– o O o –

Tipping the eyelashes with a fine scissors will increase their strength and make them grow. Exercise and good food, and a teaspoonful of Fellows's Syrup twice a day. But what does a boy want with long eyelashes?

– o O o –

Your eyes being red and eyelashes nearly absent points to something wrong constitutionally. Try cod-liver oil for months.

Now, here's something unusual:

Write to Mr. Burton, Wardour Street, Oxford Street, London, and tell him exactly the kind of eyes you want, and he will send them cheaply enough. They do not cost much; price depends on size.

Unfortunately, this almost certainly refers to a boy's query about taxidermy, rather than someone dissatisfied with the eyes he was born with.

Ears, too, could be a worry:

You had far better leave your ears alone. The efficacy of the piercing as a cure for anything is merely a vulgar superstition. Earrings are but relics of barbarism. Why not wear a ring through your nose? Would you not find the counter irritation so set up an excellent remedy for baldness?

– o O o –

BLUE EARS – The result of weak circulation. Applications no good. Brace yourself up by the bath and exercise.

– o O o –

INSTRUMENT FOR MAKING EARS LIE BACK – A pad and a bandage worn at night might do. But we fear to advise the use of any instrument.

– o O o –

If your ears 'stick out very much' we are afraid there is no remedy; as you get older it will perhaps not be so noticeable.

Here's another organ that some boys were unhappy with:

'Could you tell me what to do with my nose, it's got so red since this winter came in; could you tell me what to do with it that would keep it from getting red, and could you tell me what brought it on?' We can't: Indigestion, frostbite, or – but really you can't expect it of us this hot weather, and so we give it up!

– oOo –

You may discover a cure for 'a red nose not caused by drink' by applying to a doctor. We cannot tell you to what it should be assigned. We know nothing of nosology, and never answer medical queries. [*Interestingly, whether the Editor knew it or not, nosology is 'the systematic classification of diseases' and if this was one of Dr. Stables' replies, he almost certainly did know something of it.*]

– oOo –

No; there is no cure for an exceptionally big nose. Why, many a person would be proud of the feature. You will grow to it. Be thankful it is not a button-nose.

– oOo –

We cannot help you with the nose machine. We do not use one ourselves; and all the friends of whom we have inquired treat our question as a joke, and refuse to give a serious answer. We have been referred to the 'Proboscidean Guide,' which seems to be published somewhere in America!

– oOo –

You are surely joking! If not, we fear both you and your friend will have to be content with what nature has given you. We know of no machine for shortening noses, unless it be a chisel or a good sharp knife!

– oOo –

If you will send us a sketch of your nose, 'which is a big one and turns up at the tip,' we will see what can be done! Have you tried sandpaper?

– oOo –

RED NOSE AND FLUSHING – Your employment is rather close. Keep your windows open. Live as well as possible. Your trouble comes from a somewhat weak heart, which time and exercise alone can strengthen.

– o O o –

OSWALD and INQUISITIVE – What a pity it is that you did not give your addresses; we might then have arranged a nose exchange. What one considers an affliction the other desires; but that is the way of the world, people are never satisfied to remain as they are. Seriously, if there is anything painful about your noses you should take them to a doctor; and if there is not you should leave them alone. This answers half-a-dozen more queries on the nose.

And even if you were equipped with the right number, type, and size of moustaches, eyes, ears, and noses, there was sometimes another thing to worry about – your size:

ON THE WINGS OF THE WIND – has an objection to being called 'Two yards of pump water,' and very naturally so, we think. He will put on flesh enough when he has done growing, if he applies at once to his doctor to stop what he complains about in his second question. The cracking is owing to the joints being somewhat loose, and is not a sign of either growth or weakness.

– o O o –

How to grow your whiskers, and what to do to increase your height? Our advice is not to handicap your growth in any way; any extra weight above is prejudicial, hence always wear a very light hat, keep your hair cut very short, and post-pone raising your whisker crop until you are long enough to carry it with safety!

– o O o –

What difference there is in taste, and how manifold are people's troubles! No sooner have we soothed a youth who wants to grow tall by telling him to keep his hair cut short and reduce his top-heaviness, than you send in for information how to keep stunted and how to cultivate your head-thatch. Keep your hair as short as you can get it, and diminish your apparent height by broadening your shoulders.

– o O o –

How are you to grow - 'expence no object'? Perhaps a sea voyage, and a stay of a year or two in New South Wales would give you an inch or two extra; but the best thing is exercise, constant exercise. If you cannot be 'a great man of flesh,' be a little man of wire.

– oOo –

STOPPING GROWTH – You can't. You must continue to tower skywards and be content.

– oOo –

GLOBE writes: 'Will you kindly inform me if guano powdered is a good thing to promote growth in a boy, placed in a packet in the hollow of the foot, and whether it is injurious or not?' Can't say – we never tried it. GLOBE had better not let his schoolmates see his wise question, or they may be tempted to invent a none too-flattering nickname for him!

– oOo –

Even if boys were comfortable with their bodies, they were often worried about making the wrong impression in society:

You are in error in supposing that people in London know everything. Get rid of the notion that every one is watching you or taking the slightest interest in your dress or idiosyncrasies, and your shyness will soon evaporate. No man who is conscious of his unimportance can be 'a bore in the social sphere.'

– oOo –

Like your friends in the country, we are unable to say how you make collars shinier than when they are new. When they come from the shop they are quite shiny enough for most people. Borax added to good starch is a common mixture.

– oOo –

There is no certain remedy for creaky boots. Pour castor-oil into some shallow vessel, such as a plate, until it stands about an eighth of an inch deep, and place your boots on it for a day or two, so that the sole may absorb the oil. Castor-oil is the best thing you can put on leather to make it soft and pliable. For a stubborn pair of new boots wet them thoroughly when on, then walk in them for an hour, and then take them off and give them a copious dose of the oil rubbed well in.

– oOo –

1. Wear a piece of thin sheet india-rubber inside your hat, or some 'greaseproof' band. At the same time you will not stop the perspiration from working its way through. Benzine will clean it. 2. It is nobody's place to say 'good morning' last. That is what your point of etiquette comes to. If the master objects to your saying 'good morning' first, leave it to him to do so.

– oOo –

Keep your hat on, friend, keep it on. If you take it off to all your superiors, you will soon wear it out. You must use a little discretion in the matter.

– oOo –

We suppose that by 'Equity and Manners to Ladies' you mean a book on etiquette. But the reading of such a book would simply do you harm until you have supplied the deficiencies of your education. Learn to spell for six months, and then write again.

– oOo –

'Lancashire Lad' can obtain a book on etiquette from any London publisher. Try Dean, Ward and Lock, Warne, Routledge, etc. In all such cases 'Common sense is the best manners,' and an ounce of natural courtesy is worth a ton of the artificial variety. If you do not want to go too a party do not go, and if you are hard up for an excuse say you have got to stay at home and read the BOY'S OWN PAPER.

– oOo –

1. If your glove is on keep it on. 2. It entirely depends on your family. If they object to your slippers in the drawing-room, take them off. Existence must have a tendency to become painful in a house where special boots have to be worn for each room.

– oOo –

Raise your hat with your right hand whenever you can do so without inconvenience. You do not need to remove your glove. We leave you to discover for yourself 'the most polite way to offer a young lady your arm, and also how to gain consent to carry her umbrella.' As a rule, gentlemen who borrow umbrellas are regarded with suspicion by the ladies.

– oOo –

A gentleman walking with another who salutes a lady, whom the first does not know, ought also to lift his hat, but he need not even look towards her; indeed, he should not.

– oOo –

1. Pray take your hat off every time you see the lady. It is a graceful exercise, and it keeps the head cool. 2. It is not án invariable nor desirable custom to grunt out 'granted' when your pardon is begged; but it is considered civil to say something pleasantly as a sign that the apology is appreciated, and that there is nothing much amiss after all.

– oOo –

Take your hat off to the lady each time you meet her. The interval that has elapsed makes no difference in the mark of respect you should pay her.

– oOo –

Herr is the German equivalent of the French Monsieur and the English Mr. There is nothing particularly Jewish about it.

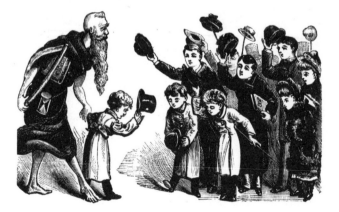

Chapter 11

===========================X===========================

'TRY AGAIN, WARRINGTON'

Crafts and hobbies for Our Boys

I̶N an era when there was no television or radio, and where 'teenagers' had not yet been invented (although there were 'teeners' in the U.S. from 1894), it's not surprising that boys occupied their time with a wide range of indoor pastimes, both at home and outdoors. The BOY'S OWN PAPER was a mine of suggestions for such hobbies, and those that involved making things often seemed to require a fully-equipped machine shop and a budget for material that would be beyond the means of many readers, however often the B.O.P. said that they were as pleased to advise a poor lad as prince. Certainly, many of the activities must have been available only to the princely end of the spectrum. One begins 'Take a leaf of gold ...' and another mentions the need for 'a voltaic battery':

> 'But we haven't got a voltaic battery,' somebody may tell me. Get
> one, then – nothing more easy. Buy one sheet of zinc about six
> inches square; a second, the same dimensions of copper. Solder
> one wire end to an extremity of the zinc-plate, the other end to
> the copper-plate – *this is your battery.* When you want it to act,
> simply immerse the two plates – they not being allowed to touch
> – in a mixture of one part to six (measure) oil of vitriol and water.

Instructions were given, sometimes over several weeks, for *The Telephone and How to make It, An Inexpensive 'Boy's Own' Writing*

*Desk, The 'Boy's Own' Dinner Gong, (*an irremediably middle-class item, that one) and even *How to Make a Violin.*

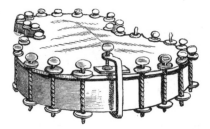

There were also instructions for an 'Aphengescope', which turned out to be a sort of overhead projector.

One article begins:

> Now that the long evenings are setting in, and knowing too that there are a large number of boys who like to make the best they can of anything they take in hand, I propose in this article to give a few practical hints showing how to build a perfect model of an inverted-cylinder direct-action engine with link-motion reversing gear, like the sketch at the beginning of this paper, which represents a type in daily use on the river and sea ...

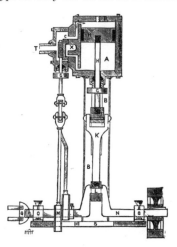

The 'sketch' looks more like the finished machine drawings in an engineering firm.

And yet, there were some suggested pastimes, decidedly weird by modern standards, which even poor boys could turn their hands to. No reader, however poor, should have much difficulty getting hold of an orange. Then, knife in hand, he could spend happy hours carving the peel into intricate shapes. If he was *really* poor, he could even eat the flesh for his supper.

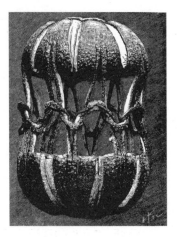

Not all the suggested hobbies were as benign as peeling an orange. Dr. Scoffern's article *Exploding Spiders and How to Make Them* contained instructions for how to make 'spiders' with a cork for a body and bristles from a blacking brush, which could then be filled with an explosive chemical mixture involving iodide of nitrogen. Once the spiders had dried, the slightest touch would make them explode. Dr. Scoffern gave readers a suggestion for where to put them:

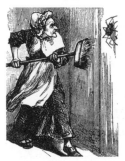

They may be set to stand on any horizontal surface; but some of the best fun I have had with them has been achieved in another manner – by attaching them to a wall or door panel by the legs with strong gum mucilage. The very first member of female humanity who sees a spider thus wandering is sure to charge the little thing full thrust with a stick or parasol, or, as it may be, a broom. You know with what result, and it is very funny.

Another article, also from the explosive pen of Dr. Scoffern, described a complicated chemical procedure for making what were called 'Pharaoh's Serpents' – small round 'eggs' which when set alight produced long snake-like protuberances, along with wafts of cyanogen, a gas which, when inhaled, according to a modern text, can lead to 'headache, dizziness, rapid pulse, nausea, vomiting, loss of consciousness, convulsions and death, depending on exposure'. Scoffern admits that the procedure can be 'a trifle dangerous', but goes on to say 'for the matter of that, it would be offensive and somewhat dangerous to ignite a lump of coal in a plate upon a table'.

The instructions begin:

> Provide yourself with an iron ladle, some sulphur, some yellow prussiate of potash – known to chemists as 'ferrocyanide of potassium' – quicksilver, nitric acid – the shop-name of which is aquafortis – filtering paper, a funnel, gum-water, a little nitre, and a bottle of distilled water.... An ingenious young fellow could do without a mortar, by crushing or rolling; he must however, by no means lay the cook's rolling-pin under contribution.

This is presumably because the tea-time scones might inadvertently become flavoured with deadly poison. Scoffern explained how the readers might have some difficulty persuading a chemist to sell them some of the ingredients, even the less harmful ones.

> 'This once happened to me, [he wrote] and as the case was amusingly provoking, I will describe it. Being in a part of London where I was not known, and needing some yellow prussiate of potash for a test, I entered a pharmaceutical chemist's shop to procure some. The governor looked at me askance, seemingly in doubt, but he handed me what I had asked for nevertheless. Before I could leave the shop he, after consulting a

list, said to me, in the blandest manner possible, 'Just let me have the parcel – I forgot to label it, as I am bound to, 'Poison'" 'You can have the parcel,' said I, but it is no more a poison than Epsom salts is a poison. When swallowed, it has pretty nearly the same effect as Epsom salts.' 'Swallow it!' ejaculated he, trembling. 'Do you mean to swallow it?' 'That is by no means my intention,' quoth I – 'it is wanted as a test.' He shook his head, returned the prussiate to his stock bottle, and would not let me have it at all.

There were some themes that recurred time and again in the *Answers to Correspondents* about hobbies and pastimes. One of them concerned what to do with used postage stamps. In the very first volume of the BOY's OWN PAPER this answer appeared:

We know of no public institution to which 'used postage stamps' will gain admittance. As to a satisfactory way of disposing of them, a good deal depends on what you may consider satisfactory. We have known of boys lining fancy boxes with them, or covering screens, etc.

With monotonous regularity the Editor was prompted to return to the theme in successive volumes:

We have already answered the question several times. We know of no one who will purchase old penny postage stamps, nor do we know of any use to which they can be put, unless it be to line fancy boxes, cover screens, etc. It is a mere popular delusion that they are of marketable value.

– oOo –

H.B. (Nottingham) writes: 'If G.E.R. wants to find a use for his old penny-stamps he might made snakes of them for the amusement of children. You get a piece of string sufficiently long to represent the intended snake, and to one end tie a cork cut in the shape of a snake's head, and then thread the stamps on the string, using halfpenny stamps as you get towards the tail.'

– oOo –

For about the hundredth time we reply that the Post-office does not buy used penny postage-stamps - nor does anybody else. You can easily prove this by offering them for sale.

– oOo –

Your used stamps are worth about eighteenpence a hundredweight. Any marine-store dealer will buy them. The 'office for their receipt' is a cruel delusion. We do our best to dissuade boys from being so foolish as to collect ...

By Volume 5 the Editor had had enough of stamps in any shape or form:

In the dim future, when we have nothing else to do, we will issue a special number containing nothing but the full particulars and prices of the four hundred stamps you inquire about. It will be so interesting to other readers!

– oOo –

The black penny English stamp is not at all rare, and can be bought now for a penny.

– oOo –

'I would be very much oblige to you if you would keep all the old stamps and envelopes for me for a week or two, and send to me by parcel delivery!' Our regret is extreme that we cannot oblige you.

Another rumour, analogous to the myth of the office that purchased used stamps, was that somewhere there was someone who would pay good money for the excretions of silkworms:

If you 'have heard of firms in London who buy silk at 21s and 10s 6d per ounce' perhaps you would not mind sending us their names. There are scores of our readers who would very much like to know them. At present we think the firms are as mythical as the used penny-postage buyers and the gold in 1864 pennies!

– oOo –

As there is no market for the silk spun by your silkworms, its quality does not matter.

– o O o –

No one will buy your silk. If you had a ton of it you might get rid of it at Lyons or Marseilles, but there is no market for it here, the trade having retired to foreign parts.

– o O o –

Give it away; there is no market for it. Many years ago there might have been, when the silk trade was very different from what it is now; but times have changed, and there is no money to be made nowadays out of keeping silkworms.

– o O o –

We cannot tell you the current price of raw silk, nor where you could dispose of so small a quantity as you are likely to have from your silkworms. To unwind the silk,

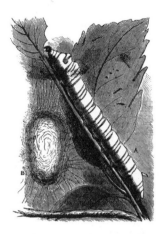

place the cocoon in a cup of warm water after removing the loose stuff. You will thus find the end, and can wind the whole upon a piece of cardboard.

– o O o –

We had an article on Silkworms in our third volume. It is an interesting occupation; but there is no getting rid of the silk, and consequently it generally ends in disappointment.

The articles on hobbies and pastimes were among the most popular:

Innumerable letters arrive with inquiries as to whether we are not going to give articles on microscopes, telescopes, and sundry instruments; also on canaries, and other song-birds; also on horses, and on silkworms; also on shorthand; also on photography; and fifty other things. To all which the answer is, 'Wait and see. We cannot take up everything at once. It is worth noticing how much we have got into a dozen numbers.'

But these articles had the unfortunate side-effect of generating a lot of correspondence from boys who misread or misunderstood the instructions, just didn't have the skills to carry them out, or wanted to contribute their own, less expert, proposals:

It is easy to see that you are a slovenly operator, from the slovenliness of your writing and orthographic errors. You state that unvulcanised rubber will not dissolve in benzoline, but merely forms a jelly. What is a jelly but a thick solution? And do you not see that by adding more benzoline you would convert the thick into a thin solution? Go on diluting with benzoline until the solution is thin enough for spreading along the edges of your silver paper with a knife. Before you so confidently affirm 'the whole thing is decidedly wrong,' be assured that you have implicitly followed instructions, and in writing again please remember the word 'balloon' has two *l*'s, and the word 'impossible' two *s*'s.

– oOo –

With your letter came one from another correspondent, who says that he has made the punt from our directions, and that it does first-rate. Why not read the instructions again? We may again touch upon boat-building presently.

– oOo –

It is probably too late now, but we have nothing to add. The description was quite accurate, and we have had many letters from lads who have made the telephone.

– oOo –

We should not at all like to go afloat in a canoe built on the plan you describe.

– oOo –

FLYING MACHINE – The instructions are all right; it is you who must have blundered somewhere. Many readers have written to express delight, amongst the latest being our artist, Mr Alfred Pearse, who says, 'I have constructed one of your flying machines, and have succeeded in making it rise quite 100 feet, travelling at the same time about 80 yards, to the delight of my little ones.'

– oOo –

We have as many articles on electricity as we shall require for some years.

– o O o –

We have already described how to make an aquarium, and we doubt if your plan would last very long.

– o O o –

A.B. says: 'Can you kindly tell me whether I could sell my fretwork, and, if so, where, and what is the general price? I have a small machine - 'The Holly' - and I have made a great many photo. frames, brackets, etc., with it, which I have hung up at home; and it is no good making any more, as we have no room for them. I should recommend any one who is going in for fretwork to have a sixpenny pantograph to enlarge or diminish his patterns. I bought one in Fleet Street about ten months ago, and I have used it nearly every day since.' For the information of A.B. and many other correspondents, does any one know where fretwork can be disposed of at a reasonable rate?

– o O o –

It is impossible to describe it without illustrations and diagrams, but we shall probably publish an article on fancy netting one of these days.

– o O o –

Artificial flowers can be made from potatoes and turnips, but the result is generally but a very poor imitation of beautiful objects.

– o O o –

Working human hair into initials, etc., is a long and tedious process. You had better consult some accomplished female friend.

– o O o –

For sticking in scraps and other small pasting jobs, you will scarcely get a better thing than Field and Tuer's 'Stickphast Office Paste,' which sells at a shilling per pot.

– o O o –

We are indeed glad to hear that you have 'succeeded in making a very fair and good-toned violin' from our articles, as we must confess that it is by no means an easy thing to do. Violin-making requires much patience and ingenuity.

– o O o –

If you can get good violins for 18s. you had better buy all the man has at the price, and you will soon make your fortune. You cannot buy much of an instrument under ordinary circumstances for less than fifty shillings.

– oOo –

Give about fifty shillings for a good violin to some respectable musical instrument seller, and bring your wanderings to brokers' shops in search of genuine Stradivarii to a sudden close. A good bow will cost you half a guinea.

– oOo –

You may have a genuine instrument, but if the label is spelt as you spell it, it must be a forgery. Perhaps you have a copy, and have misread. An expert like Mr Hart of Wardour Street could tell you; but Cremona violins are like old masters - their whereabouts are mostly well known and registered by those interested in selling them.

– oOo –

The wires for a telephone need not run in a straight line. You can turn them about as much as you please, provided you keep them insulated. A small electric alarm-bell might cost you five shillings.

– oOo –

Yours was a very ordinary performance. The delicacy of present object-mounting is something marvellous. At one of the recent meetings of the Quekett, Mr. E.T. Newton exhibited the head of a cockroach which he had sliced into no less than thirty two pieces. Of the section on each slide he had made a cardboard model of the size it appeared through the microscope, and on each piece of cardboard he had accurately drawn and coloured an exact reproduction of the original - of course, on the enlarged scale. The thirty-two pieces of cardboard, when placed side by side, fitted exactly, and formed a huge model of the cockroach's head, correct in every particular.

– oOo –

We fear that Edison's electric pen is too mechanically delicate for a boy's home manufacture.

– oOo –

Your idea is well known to the Aeronautical Society. The plan is as old as the French Revolution, and has always failed for the lack of a sufficiently light motor. Like ninety-nine hundredths of our modern inventors, you have been forestalled.

– o O o –

P. WARRINGTON – There is evidently 'something stupid' somewhere. It may be in the plate, but we do not think so. Many other readers seem to have made the model ship, judging from the letters which reach us. LIMERICK, for instance, writes to-day: 'I have succeeded in putting it together. It is a very pretty ornament, and is very much admired by all my friends; few could believe it was paper till they looked closely at it.' Try again, Warrington!

– o O o –

The difficulty of cleaning your revolver can be got over by giving it away before it gets dirty.

– o O o –

Potatoes boiled in sulphuric acid are said to be turned into artificial meerschaum, but it is not safe to put it in your mouth. Some of the artificial ivory is said to be so made. You carve the pattern first, and then harden it.

– o O o –

Quite correct - if you mean the banjo. We will have a turn at the banjo in the good time coming.

– o O o –

You can get such books from any magical warehouse.

– o O o –

E. A. – We are much obliged to you for sending us from Australia the particulars of your invention for propelling balloons; but, alas! the idea of generating gas under pressure, and using it directly in a jet, and indirectly in an engine, has been tried before. The firework notion is too crude. What size rocket do you think you would require to drive a balloon against a breeze for a dozen miles or so? *[E.A. was presumably discouraged from developing an idea which Frank Whittle used as the basis for the jet engine fifty years later.]*

– o O o –

For gas-stoves for laboratory purposes you could not do better than apply to Mr. Fletcher, Warrington. He is the great authority on gas as a fuel. Gas fires are much used in the arts. What do you think of a gas flame forty feet long, and only half an inch thick?

– o O o –

Fireproof the document. Soak it in a strong solution of alum. You can throw paper on the fire when thus treated, and it will not be in the least damaged.

– oOo –

If you have not sufficient time to play 'a bango or a cordien or a concertina,' your chance of musical proficiency is almost hopeless. Perhaps the tambourine or the bones might suit you, though it is not an easy thing to play the bones properly.

– oOo –

One of the prize-winners in our recent competition informs us that hoofs can be purchased from any tripe-shop at a penny per pair.

– oOo –

The three-ply wood for fret-cutting is made by Mr. J.H. Skinner, of East Dereham, Norfolk. The centre layer runs the opposite way of the grain to the others. The prices per square foot are sixpence for an eighth of an inch thick, sevenpence for three-sixteenths of an inch, and eight-pence for a quarter-inch. This is for walnut, mahogany, and brown oak; other woods cost fivepence, sixpence, and sevenpence.

– oOo –

You procure a cocoanut costing threepence, and a lathe and tools costing five pounds; and with these, after much practice, you may succeed in making a farthing ring. Could you not employ your time more profitably?

– oOo –

The title of the article was 'How to Make an Astronomical Telescope,' and an astronomical telescope is what you have made. All astro-nomical telescopes make things appear upside down. The telescope does not bring things nearer to you; it magnifies them, and conse-quently makes them appear near.

– oOo –

The 'spirits' used in the glasses that give forth their sounds under the fingers of the street musician are simply water. Any fluid will do, and the instrument will keep tune for a long time providing you do not play it in a shower of rain.

– oOo –

Unscrew the burner and turn the gas full on into the balloon, which you should hold above it. Fill it much the same as you would a bladder with a tobacco-pipe.

– oOo –

A correspondent writes from Hereford: 'I have made a cardboard engine according to directions given in B.O.P. I sent it to the Church of England Temperance Society's Industrial and Art Exhibition which was held here, when it gained a first-prize of 7s. 6d. I was twelve years old last May.'

– oOo –

The coating of indiarubber is too thin, but you will spoil your mackintosh if you attempt to thicken it.

– oOo –

Get Macmillan's Shilling Primer of Electricity. It is pure waste of time making scientific apparatus unless you know what you are doing.

– oOo –

You cannot get a skull white that has been buried some time. It is indelibly stained.

– oOo –

DIARY (Sir B. Fandango, S.A.) – The best use to which you can put a diary is to make it an index of the books you read. Write on one side of the paper only. Every day make a full index (not in alphabetical order) of whatever you have read, be it the Bible or any book, but keep the entries for each book separate. At the close of the year cut your diary up into slips, sort these out into their books, arrange them in alphabetical order, and make a fair copy. You will thus get a series of indexes of every book you have read, which will be of lasting value to you through life. For ordinary diaries that begin very full in January, and dwindle down to 'took a walk' in April, we have but the very slightest commendation.

– oOo –

Hopeless. A good lantern will cost you two or three guineas; what can you expect for elevenpence? Get a new lamp, new lenses, and a new case. A good reflector behind the present lamp might help you.

– oOo –

You can make cork shoes but you cannot walk on water with them.

– oOo –

You require a great deal more power than you can get out of your clockwork. You will never get screws and paddlewheels to support and drive a box through the air if you have only got a spring to work them with. The invention has been frequently tried before and failed, owing to the want of a sufficiently light motor.

– oOo –

We have answered this question a dozen times, and have taken to putting such letters in the waste-paper-basket at once. There never was any gold in the 1864 pennies, and it is simply impossible that there could be. The Mint is not a small kitchen with all the cooking going on in one place. The copper is coined in one wing of the building, the silver and gold in the other, with quite different appliances, and in quite a different way. The statement is a baseless falsehood, originally started as a practical joke on a poor simpleton who was induced to waste his money by buying up the coppers supplied him by the joker.

– oOo –

A remarkable display of fatuousness. The indiarubber cement has been known for years, and is used by the gallon every day. Try again. You have got as far as the jelly, now get as far as the glue. You can substitute benzine or bisulphide of carbon if you please.

– oOo –

Please do not send us coins to name or value. The risk of their being lost is great, and we do not hold ourselves responsible for their safety. If you want them named or valued take them to the curator of your local museum. As a rule you may take it for granted that the coin is worth a little less than the metal of which you think it is made, and that nine-tenths of the coins in your collection are practically valueless.

– oOo –

Attend science classes in electricity and magnetism. Every town has them during the winter months, and the fees are almost nominal. It is pure waste of time to play with apparatus which you evidently don't understand.

Just occasionally, the Editor displayed a twinkle of boyish mischief in his replies:

You can tan model-boat sails by boiling them in the coffee-pot – a *deed of darkness often done but seldom mentioned.* The best plan is to steep them in a solution of oak bark, of which a pennyworth - bark or solution - will go a long way.

But for the most part, in a magazine that was based on Christian principles, it's not surprising that the Editor felt obliged from time to time to issue a sharp reprimand, faced with the evidence in some of the letters of the innate wickedness of boys, and he came down heavily on any lapse from high moral standards:

The object of a debating society is to bring out your own ideas on the subject under discussion, and under no circumstances will we be parties to a scheme which impels you to write to us to supply you with thoughts and facts at the expense of your schoolfellows.

– oOo –

We cannot here describe the manufacture of whisky. You will become a naturalist more rapidly by leaving off the whisky.

– oOo –

The easiest way to make a blowpipe is to buy two or three ounces of glass tubing from the nearest druggist's, and to use as darts large darning needles wrapped round with worsted. If, instead of blowpipes, you were to call them 'puff and darts,' you would find them on sale at nearly every toyshop, target and all complete. The poisoned darts of the Macoushie are of course not obtainable.

– oOo –

We never answer such questions. There would soon be a vacancy for a 'Boys Own Coroner' if we did. you had better insure your life if you purpose continuing such a line of inquiry.

– oOo –

You had better not try tricks with fire, much less with molten lead. The conjurors have special ways of protecting themselves ...

– oOo –

We do not know of anything that will erase ink from postage stamps; and if we did we should not divulge it!

– oOo –

We cannot, even on receipt of 'stamp and address' undertake to send you a 'sectioned drawing of a gas-meter'.

– oOo –

You have gone quite far enough in your experiments with phosphorous; if you attempt more you will probably have an accident.

– oOo –

We do not care to give recipes for making gunpowder. What would your parents say to us?

– oOo –

We do not know of any gun manufacturers in want of an apprentice ...

– oOo –

You would be liable to imprisonment if captured, but your friends could claim your clothes and chest.

– oOo –

You must have a licence for guns and pistols of all kinds, and with

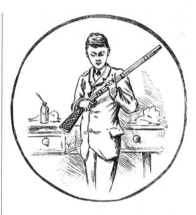

the sort you mention an Accidental Insurance policy is valuable, as the pistol has a reputation for occasionally going off at the wrong end.

– oOo –

You must have a licence for a gun, no matter what you shoot with it. It is the gun that is licensed, not the thing you shoot at.

– oOo –

We cannot say if the songs you mention are copyright; probably they are. You should be very careful not to sing any song in public, even for the best of purposes, without having first obtained the written permission of the person to whom its copyright belongs. There are one or two lawyers in London who make it their business to ferret out and hush up for a consideration every petty infringement of the copyright of musical pieces at even the obscurest of entertainments.

– o O o –

Ask your father, schoolmaster, or some gentleman friend to get it for you. No chemist is likely to sell such a deadly poison as prussic acid to boys.

– o O o –

The only way we can suggest for you to find out where your friend is buried is for you to advertise in the London morning papers.

– o O o –

We have never taken any interest in matters connected with the turf, and questions concerning its eccentricities are promptly consigned to our waste-paper basket.

– o O o –

The marriage certificate is merely a copy of the record of the marriage, and has no value in itself. The record is the important thing; it is kept at the place where the ceremony was performed, and in these days is not likely to be lost.

The 'gentleman' who mislaid the marriage certificate, and married again on the strength of the loss, has been rather premature, as he will find to his cost when steps are taken against him.

– o O o –

You are liable to a heavy penalty for not having the boy's birth registered, and it will be enforced unless you are very careful. Consult some minister or doctor.

– o O o –

You can hardly expect us to give a series of articles on lock-picking ...

– o O o –

Ask your medical man to procure some for you. Any qualified surgeon or general practitioner can obtain it, but we warned you in our pages that druggists are very cautious about selling so deadly a poison.

– o O o –

The coolness of your request is quite refreshing. We wonder what our contributors will say when they hear that 'an admiring correspondent' is anxious to have some rejected MSS. that have been sent to us 'by different persons,' that he can publish them gratuitously in his school magazine! We beg to decline, with thanks, of course. Why not write all the paper yourself? You are quite equal to it, we can assure you.

– o O o –

There are many varieties of gunpowder, and none of them are allowed to be made by private persons.

– o O o –

The marks are all right and the maker is well known; but we never guarantee firearms, or encourage our readers to play with them. The marks look so mysterious because you have looked at them upside down.

– o O o –

It looks suspiciously like an examination question, and such queries we do not answer. However, we will give you a hint. The Lords Appellant 'flourished' in the reign of Richard II.

– o O o –

You must withdraw your application, and refrain from applying again for a situation in which a certificate is required. No crueller wrong can be done a child than the refusal to comply with the law as to the registration of its birth, etc. Your parents are liable to a fine for their neglect, to say nothing of the injustice they have done you.

– o O o –

For lightning-paper... take the very greatest care all through, as the slightest slip or mistake may necessitate a doctor's bill, if not a coroner's inquest. Hence all such matters are best not dabbled in by amateurs.

– o O o –

We gave articles on peculiar punishments in the fifth volume.

– o O o –

We do not answer such queries. It would be impossible to do so justly without knowing all the circumstances. You had better consult a respectable solicitor.

– o O o –

We have heard of flouring people's pillows, but we never knew any good come of it. Such fun soon becomes stale. Practical jokes generally end in practical unpleasantness.

– o O o –

You are not allowed to make explosives without a licence from the Home Office. When you have got the licence, and had your buildings passed by the inspector, we will tell you how to set to work.

– o O o –

If you carry firearms you must have a licence. It does not matter what they are or what they are called, or what is their size or weight, or which end goes off when you fire!

– o O o –

Even in these days you hear of men 'selling' their wives, but such things are not 'customs.' In no time in this country has it been legal to do such a thing, or has the transfer been recognised; and in no time has the practice ever been indulged in except by the lowest of the low.

– o O o –

If a boy breaks a window he should pay for the damage. The streets are not for the spinning of whiptops, but for traffic; and if you choose to spin whiptops in the street near windows 'which have no protection' you must take the consequences. Is it reasonable to suppose that the tradesman ought to fit his windows with somebody's 'whiptop protector' to suit your peculiar idiosyncrasy?

– o O o –

There is no such sale of Government arms at present.

– o O o –

The 'few boys of Liverpool' should be informed that under the last Explosives Act the making of fireworks by amateurs is against the law, and may bring them into unpleasant communication with the police. All 'explosives' have now to be manufactured on registered premises. The reason that no articles on fireworks now appear in the paper is that some time ago we received a call from one of the Government inspectors, who explained to us the bearing of the new law on such apparently trivial matters. If the boys want fireworks they must buy them ready-made, or run the risk of heavy penalties.

– o O o –

Whisky, gin, rum, brandy, etc., are the best things in the world for the inside of a *rat's hole*, and oatmeal-porridge the best thing on earth for a boy's inside. But make 'them' thick, and do not boil them more than five minutes!

– o O o –

You have no right to use a catapult in a road and the policeman was doing you a service in taking it away from you.

– o O o –

If your question be a conundrum, we give it up. If you mean seriously that you lost your master's moneys, we do not understand how you could even raise a question as to legality. An honourable boy would have paid back the sum so lost as soon as he could, without such a thought occurring to him.

– o O o –

We cannot occupy our space with seditious matter.

– o O o –

Ridiculous! The sanitary authorities would soon interfere if a creditor attempted to detain a corpse until the dead man's debts were paid.

– o O o –

If the boy next door carries out his threat of killing your pigeons when trespassing, the law can make him pay full value and costs. At the same time he can hold you good for injury done to his crops, which doubtless are very extensive!

– o O o –

If you commit a murder you will certainly be hanged for it, no matter how long you hide, or how much you confess; and we should advise you to refrain from thinking of such things, and asking questions about them, though you may be in ever so great a hurry.

'SUNKEN SPORULES BECOME MIXED'
Riddles wrapped in enigmas

The Editor often pointed out that the B.O.P. only published answers that would be of interest to other boys. COBBLES, for example, was told:

> What interest can there be to our readers in our opinion of your handwriting? If you did not think it exquisite you would not send it to us to admire. The information in these columns is not for the sole benefit of the questioner, but for that of our readers in general.

This was not strictly true – there were some answers which could not be of interest to anyone since the original query was undetectable. A reply like 'All about it before long' would be mildly interesting to 'N.H.S.' who would have to look in future issues for articles about the subject of his query, but to 'readers in general' it would be impenetrable.

Here's a selection of 'mystery' answers. Some, I suppose, are only mysterious to people (like me) who don't know what jack-lines or vangs are. The meaning of others is likely to remain hidden until the end of time.

1. Arranged. 2. Impossible to say without seeing the egg. 3. Not now. 4. You had better buy one, but a piece of mackintosh properly folded and strapped does just as well. 5. Any optician's. They are nearly all made at the same place.

– o O o –

We have no recipe just at hand for dressing jack-lines.

– o O o –

Very possibly, but you must not be in too great a hurry, as there are many tastes to gratify.

– o O o –

We never before heard of 'bang hops' consequently we cannot tell you how to make them.

– o O o –

1. For small quantities of circulars and so forth. 2. Walk on. 3. Not unless you have been introduced. 4. No. 5. On the right hand. 6. Allowable. Why not buy a book? You can get one for a shilling. 7. Wherever you like, and whichever you please.

– o O o –

It would be cheaper to buy the glass density balls at the dealers. 2. Sunken sporules become mixed, and therefore visible. Splashing water into the vessel will mostly clarify it.

– o O o –

Certainly not, because the single strand has to wind round three times in order to made a grummet. The following is a very good proportion to work by: – Four-stranded rope, to make a three-stranded strop for a block or a yard. Three times the round of the block or yard, three times the round of the thimble. Then allow sufficient length to splice it, which you will find will be about six times the round of the

rope. With three-stranded rope you require three times the round of the yard, three times the round of the thimble, and three times the round of the rope, then allow six times the round of the rope for splicing. If you only took three times the diameter, you would be all adrift.

– o O o –

In such a matter you had better consult your friends, and if possible you might make inquiries personally at some firm of tea-brokers.

– o O o –

Yes, as nearly as possible.

– o O o –

Once is enough.

– o O o –

We did not mean the X.Y., and we regret there was anything in the context to lead you to think so. Read our remarks again, and you will see that you have been defending what we never attacked.

– o O o –

1. Thanks for the suggestion. 2. About a couple of pounds. 3. Arranged. 4. Our remarks were

principally directed against the custom amongst some lads of sitting about without their clothes and not taking to the water as soon as ready. 5. See our articles on Gymnastics. 6. No.

– o O o –

Downing Street, Whitehall, S.W. Do you want him to send you a postcard?

– o O o –

Rub it over well with a piece of indiarubber, and write with blue-black ink.

– o O o –

1. Work with your palms upwards. 2. It does them no harm.

– o O o –

No; and surely you can see why. We have found our size most suitable.

– o O o –

There is no necessity for the procedure you recommend if the gut be crushed between the teeth for three-eighths of an inch of its extreme end. If the whipping-silk be well-waxed, evenly bound, and securely tied, even the crushing is not an absolute necessity. Thanks for your suggestion, however.

1. The mysterious 'instrument' is a policeman's staff. 2. Buy one for sixpence; it will save a lot of description. 3. In prison, at Dartmoor and elsewhere in this country. There is no transportation nowadays; the colonies did not appreciate our supplying them with criminal leaven.

– o O o –

Powdered fluor is fluor powdered. Try another shop, unless by mistake you asked the question of the errand-boy. Did you never hear of Blue John?

– o O o –

You can get an Oeolipile at most chemical-appliance shops. You have not got its description quite right, but the thing is well known.

– o O o –

By the 'sheet ropes of the gaff of a three-master's spanker' we suppose you mean the 'vangs.' The 'topping lift' joins the ends of the gaff and the spanker-boom.

– o O o –

We regret that your feelings should have been hurt by the picture of the skinning of the chum. The phrase, however, is one far more terse and intelligible to the majority of our readers than anything you can suggest. Your remarks are evidently penned in ignorance of the fact that all things are progressive. In language, the colloquial of one century is the classical of the next. Even your own letter opens with an expression that fifty years ago was slang of the vulgarest. If primitive man had never gone beyond the words he found in his dictionary, where in the name of wonder should we be?

– o O o –

You could make the bottom and corners of wood, and cover them with Portland cement.

– o O o –

We regret that we are unable to inform you in what year the whole of the British foreign possessions were governed by the natives of Cork. Perhaps some county Cork lad can oblige.

– o O o –

We have no views on Danish butter. Is it a mystery?

– o O o –

Say 'carpets beaten,' and avoid all chance of dispute.

Circumstances have occurred which render it unadvisable to enter into correspondence with strangers on school matters, and you must trust for information to what has been printed in 'Tom Brown's Schooldays' and other such works.

– o O o –

It is desirable that you should obtain your correspondent through your friends, and not through the public press. There are certain reasons for this which your father or minister may explain to you.

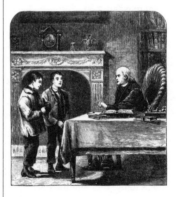

– o O o –

A 'faculty' vault is one that can be opened for burials on application to the faculty of the diocese. By the Intramural Burials Act many of the graveyards were closed, but a few of these vaults exist which can be used on special application.

– o O o –

We are obliged to you for your sketch of the wall-paper. The restless effect is obvious enough. If you are passing along the south side of Gordon Square you will notice the steps of a doctor's house in which the tiles have been so arranged as to make them seem on the move.

– o O o –

Steam it; that is the only plan, and that may fail.

– o O o –

The shots were fired by the balloonists. Had it been otherwise the sentence would have been finished.

– o O o –

Messrs. Mather and Co., of Farringdon Road, used at one time to supply the shouldered chipboxes, but we are informed that they have now ceased to do so, owing to the very limited demand. They offer, however, to import them specially for any customer who will take £15 worth! Try the shouldered cardboard boxes. You

ought to be able to procure them without difficulty, and they will answer just as well.

– o O o –

Certainly it is of value if in quantities that pay working. There are fuller's-earth works at Nutfield in Surrey, a mile or two eastward of Redhill station.

– o O o –

The system is well known, and the books can be obtained through any bookseller. There are several opposition systems. 'The art is not more generally used' because the apparatus occasionally collapses.

– o O o –

1. Try at an umbrella manufacturer's. 2. With only one or two exceptions there are no *Noctuae* on the wing in May. Therefore it is useless to sugar.

– o O o –

It does not look promising, but you might use asbestos, obtainable from the company opposite the 'Times' office in Queen Victoria Street; or even pumice, or flowerpot, or brick. All of these things are porous, and will stand heat.

– o O o –

You cannot restrict a word to its original meaning in this hurried, loosely-thinking world. You would put us in never-ending strife with our contributors. And why? - or, rather, how? However, thanks.

– o O o –

On no account attempt to drive a boat with a sheet-tin boiler. Refer to our back numbers.

– o O o –

Exactly; and the question emanated from Colney Hatch. If you multiply a gallon of pitch by a quart of periwinkles, what is the result?

– o O o –

Never heard that before. How can this be said to be of interest to other boys?

– o O o –

The tale about blowing into a camel to raise the wind is a 'romance of the Sahara.'

– o O o –

1. One pair of doors is enough for the space you name. 2. No; only an expert could tell. 3. You feed rightly. 4. Yes.

– o O o –

Unnatural indeed. Do not try any such tricks. Your friend is a *stultus*.

– o O o –

What do you mean by 'Hoove's cattle have the hoove after a blow-out.' We did not know boys did.

– o O o –

We are unaware of any record of the man who made the first box to keep money in with a hole in the middle.

– o O o –

The back-handed one is best for book-keeping, but it does not matter much.

Chapter 12

=====================================X=====================================

'FOR BOYS, NOT BY THEM'

Competition and creativity

O NE back-handed tribute to the high quality of the BOY's OWN PAPER was the fact that boys were sometimes tempted to plagiarise its contents, although why they were stupid enough to ask the Editor for permission is difficult to fathom:

We certainly will not give permission for you to take stories from this paper and send them in to win prizes from another paper.

– oOo –

Our stories and articles are all copyright, and we do not allow them to be sent by readers for publication in other journals to 'win prizes.'

– oOo –

We decidedly object to your taking one of our stories and sending it in for a prize in a competition in another journal. We fail, however, to see what good it would do you, as it would be recognised immediately.

Some years later, an incident of plagiarism was to show that it *was* possible to fool even the B.O.P. itself. In the 1920s, a twelve-year-old reader of the BOY's OWN PAPER copied out a poem called *His Requiem*, which began:

> Nobody cared a bit, folks said,
> When that wicked old man at the farm lay dead ...

The boy sold it to the *Western Mail* for ten shillings, and emboldened by his success he copied another poem, called *The Second Best,* from a volume of the B.O.P. published seventeen years earlier, and sent it to – the BOY'S OWN PAPER. Far from being 'recognised immediately' it was published in February, 1927. The boy was to move on and write his own poetry, showing that he could produce far better work than the two B.O.P. poets. His name was Dylan Thomas.

In the 1880s, the magazine published details of an incident which sounded suspiciously like professional plagiarism nipped in the bud, or rather after the fruit had dropped. It concerned a serial story called *Harry Treverton,* 'by Lady Broome', which had run from October to December, 1887.

While the serial was in full flow, someone had sent the B.O.P. a cutting from an Australian newspaper which said:

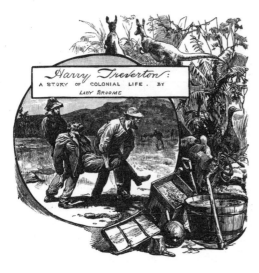

A new aspirant for literary fame has appeared in the person of Mr. W. H. Timperley, Superintendent of Rottnest Island. 'Far from the madding crowd,' he has devoted the leisure won from his official duties on his island home to the writing of a West Australian story. It is entitled 'Harry Treverton' and has advanced so far beyond the merely initial stage as to have been actually accepted by a

publisher, and it is now in the press. It is to be published in the
BOY'S OWN PAPER, as a serial story, and the opening chapters will
probably appear in the number of that periodical for the present
month, which will arrive here about the end of November.'

So was 'Lady Broome' a pseudonym or did she really exist?
Lady Broome turned out to be the wife of the Governor of Western
Australia, and she explained apologetically to the B.O.P. in a letter
which arrived about the same time: 'I did not wish to reclaim the
authorship, but only to appear as the editor of the tale. It is written
by a Mr. W. H. Timperley, a very valued colonist, at present
Superintendent of Rottnest Island, and for many years an Inspector
of Police in Western Australia. He supplied the rough draft of the
material, drawn from his own experience and knowledge, and I
undertook to present it in a readable form.' So that's all right then.

Serial stories like *Harry Temperley, Nearly Eaten,* and
Raymond Frézols: A Strange Story of Pluck, Pith and Peradventure,
often pitted good against evil in a series of cliff-hanging episodes
which sometimes lasted six months. Good always triumphed, but
for the serials to work, evil had to be portrayed in a convincingly
realistic light, which occasionally led to criticisms from parents.
Characteristically, the Editor was robust in his defence and used
his reply to one criticism to emphasise the Christian credentials of
the B.O.P.:

A correspondent having written to complain about 'My Doggie
and I,' apparently because, and simply because, there were
some 'rough characters' in it, and also to condemn the illustrations for making a burglar look like one (which of course was
the precise object of the artist, unless he had deliberately sacri-
ficed truth as well as common sense, and thus stultified the
noble lessons it was the design of the story to teach), we
forwarded the complaint to Mr. Ballantyne, who writes: 'It

grieves me deeply to find that "My Doggie," which I had earnestly hoped would do good, has given offence in some quarters. One of my chief aims in the story is to show the blessed influence of *love*, in drawing light, careless, and depraved hearts away from sin towards Jesus, the Saviour from sin. In attempting this I have had to contrast coarse, vulgar, and bad characters with those that are good, tender, and true. Surely the most sensitive of your readers must admit that it is impossible to exhibit

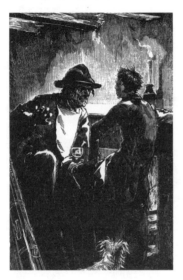

such a contrast without a faithful portraiture of both characters. A villain must of necessity speak, look, and act as a villain if he is to appear on the stage at all.' By the same post came a second letter, from an equally confident and authoritative correspondent, extolling 'Doggie,' but complaining of the 'Watch' story [*The Adventures of a Three-Guinea Watch*, by Talbot Baines Reed], on precisely similar grounds. The author of the 'Watch' (who is the son of Sir Charles Reed, Chairman of the London School Board) writes: 'The great strength of the BOY'S OWN PAPER (which is far away the healthiest and manliest I know) seems to me to lie in its high moral and religious tone,' – a tone which it was the special object of his story to maintain and strengthen. It would almost seem as though our correspondents wrote without having really read what they complained of. To merely glance at but one picture or chapter, and then, finding it to contain a ruffian or dissipated youth, to therefore conclude that the story is 'low,' or even not all that the most sensitive Christian

could desire, would seem still more irrational than the action of
the Irishman who is reputed to have brought a single brick to
enable a purchaser to judge of the value of his house!

Within hours of this defence of its serials appearing in the
shops, B.O.P.'s readers young and old, rushed to add their whole-
hearted support, and the Editor felt compelled to return to the fray
in the *Answers to Correspondents* column:

All our kind correspondents - and they are far too numerous to
particularise – who have written to us endorsing our note on this
subject in No. 114 are heartily thanked. We rejoice to see that
amongst the writers are the heads of some of the largest private
and public schools, and others occupying official positions. Such
spontaneous testimony, coming from such quarters, to the high
appreciation in which the BOY'S OWN PAPER is held, and as to
the good it is doing, cannot but encourage and strengthen us in
our responsible labours. Of course we did not expect to please all,
and the unanimity of our correspondents is therefore all the
more gratifying. One writer, who 'takes forty-three copies of the
BOY'S OWN PAPER for his Sunday-school,' further shows that he
has the 'success of the paper wholly at heart,' by sending us
something for our Note Book. Another correspondent writes
from a Birkenhead school, in which 'upwards of 200 boys take in
the paper.' The head of a Dartford grammar-school writes: 'As a
constant reader of the "Christian" as well as of the BOY'S OWN
PAPER, I am so far qualified to give an opinion on both. I
certainly would not place the former indiscriminately in the
hands of my pupils . . . but the latter must change its character
before I hesitate to permit its freest circulation, or cease to delight
in its proving so great an attraction for boys.'

The confidence in its own policies that underpinned the B.O.P.'s
responses to criticism showed that it knew who its readers were

and what they would enjoy, while sticking firmly to its principles. And the readers were an intelligent lot, who did not need to be talked down to or spoon-fed, partly – obviously – because they were at good schools. One gauge of the readership's acumen was in the humour that was put before them, some of which even reads amusingly today:

'I've just looked in to see if you are doing well,' as the cook said to the lobster, when she lifted up the saucepan lid.

– o O o –

A little boy put a lighted match into a nearly empty powder keg to see what would happen. He will not do so again, as his curiosity is satisfied; but the girl who sits next to him in school thinks he looked better with his nose on.

– o O o –

Why should railway travellers invariably avoid the 12.50 train? Because it would be 10 to 1 if they caught it.

– o O o –

It was an examination in Household Economy. 'Describe fully the method you would adopt for the preparation of beef-tea.' 'Buy a pot of Liebig's extract of beef, and rigidly follow the directions on the tin.'

– o O o –

We have all heard of the boy who, on being asked who signed Magna Charta, replied 'Please, sir, I didn't.' I never until recently heard the examiner's remark in continuation. Seeing that he had unintentionally frightened the urchin, he said, in a kindly tone, 'My dear boy, there was nothing wrong in signing it; on the contrary, it was an act meriting great praise.' Whereupon a youngster shouted out, 'Please sir, I done it! I done it by myself!'

– o O o –

'Cheek,' and an attempt to score off his adversary, is generally the cause of the most ludicrous replies given by the examinee. 'Perhaps you can quote a text,' a long-suffering examiner said to a man who showed a most hopeless state of ignorance. 'No, I don't think I can,' was the answer. 'But try,' said the examiner. After considerable reflection the undergraduate said he did know one: 'Judas went and hanged himself.' 'Quite right,' said the examiner approvingly. 'Can you mention another?' The student gazed steadily at his persecutor for a few seconds, and then replied, 'Go thou and do likewise.'

(Even these were not to everyone's taste:

No; we must remember we have readers who *can* appreciate jokes. We cannot delete them all for the sake of 'George Thompson, Perth.')

The fact that the readers of the B.O.P. could enjoy its writings and illustrations with some degree of sophistication unfortunately led some of them to believe they could produce as good material themselves, which led in the *Correspondence* columns to some of the strongest rebuffs from the Editor, who, as we've seen, didn't often pull his punches:

If the Boys Own Paper is written *for* boys, it is not written *by* them, only the highest available talent in the various departments being employed. Such contributions as yours, therefore, are of no manner of use.

– o O o –

As you are so pressing for us to be candid we will be so. We only looked at one page, and we can assure you that you are not a shining light at verse. Your twinkle is but feeble, and occasionally drops into darkness – in fact, the light fails owing to the unsatisfactory condition of the meter. Apart from the anachronism, blunderbuss is not admissible as a rhyme to Columbus.

– o O o –

Do not send the long poem. There are showers of volunteered verses by every post.

– o O o –

The poetical recollections of the Eildon Hills would interest a very small proportion of our readers. We admire the writer's patriotic feeling if not his poetic skill, and we hope his love of the old Tweedside home will never be lost.

– oOo –

If the tales are really worth publishing, you will probably, in time, find editors willing to take them. If they have no special merits, it will be far cheaper and better to burn them than to attempt publication on your own account.

– oOo –

We really cannot undertake to read the verses of amateur poets, or to express, either here or through the post, our opinion as to their merits. Verses sent to us for publication will, if found suitable and we have the space, be inserted; if not, at once destroyed, unless accompanied by a properly addressed and stamped envelope. In no case can we enter into explanations about them, as they reach us by basketfuls.

– oOo –

It is of no manner of use sending such amateur productions. What-ever other papers may do, our space is far too valuable to be given up to third or fourth-rate stories.

– oOo –

The Poet Laureateship, so far as salary goes, is worth £300 a year, but its value as an advertisement is something considerable. 'Go in for it' by all means. There is no vacancy at present, but – no matter! By the bye, do not trouble to improve your spelling, it would decrease your stock of rhymes.

– oOo –

Your case is hopeless, W.W.! Stick to prose. Poets, like other mortals, go to school, and there, we suppose, they learn their punctuation. But you will never become laureate after a start like yours – 'Please can you tell me weather Poets put their own stops in, or weather the printer puts them in. And if the poet puts them in, how does he acquire the knowl-edge to do it?' Perhaps Mr. Tennyson will oblige.

– oOo –

We can do nothing with 'the poetry that might come in useful somewhere.' Did you ever read Gray's Elegy on the same subject?

– oOo –

We will have another competition in picture-describing later on. Please send us no more MSS., we cannot use them. Were you the sole survivor who hid himself in the sea-chest when the mate fired his pistol into the magazine and blew the short-sworded pirate and co. into smithereens?

– oOo –

Unless we read the story we cannot say, and unless it is written on one side of the paper only we will not read it. Under the circumstances we think it better to decline. Why you should take the trouble to put yourself entirely beyond hope is to us inexplicable. A moment's thought would show you that, written on both sides of the paper, the copy becomes very troublesome if not useless for printers.

– oOo –

MILTON – Thanks – many thanks. But we have read enough. Do not trust the valuable MS. to the post. The cost of carriage would be considerable, and the 'poem' is so

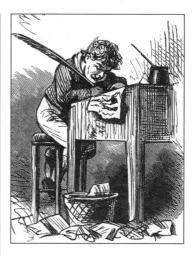

weak in its feet that our readers might not like to see it toddling over forty pages. The opening stanza is sufficient to give you the 'fame' you speak of:-

> "Tis placid eve, and the
>   circumambulatory moon,
> Doth gaze on us like a cherubim
>   in its sphere,
> Sir Ralph the Rover says that he
>   will be soon
> Amongst his family here.'

– oOo –

THE POETS OF THE FUTURE ask, 'Are the poems you get from other boys anything like ours?' Unfortunately in many cases they are! 'The Poets of the Future' seem to fancy that verse is another name for nonsense cut up into short lengths. We can *not* use such verses.

– o O o –

Our opinion is the same as that of your relatives. Please send us no more. You have evidently mistaken your gifts.

– o O o –

We are not in want of any such story. Pray do not send the MS.

– o O o –

Such amateur verses are of no manner of use to us.

– o O o –

Neither the 'drawings' nor the 'verses' will be inserted. Send them to another paper. They are much too 'funny' for us; very much too much, in fact.

– o O o –

Never send verses to magazines unless you possess independent means. It is only very rarely indeed that payment is made for such contributions. And, to speak frankly, you are wasting your time, as you evidently fail to understand the first principles of versification.

– o O o –

'But still we take no notice though they are on Death's rim!' What is 'Death's rim'? Is it the only rhyme to dim you could find? We do not remember to have heard it before. Your imagination must be somewhat remarkable. You only want two things to be a poet – sense and sound – and at present you have neither.

– o O o –

Pray do not trouble to send us the translations. We should have no space for them for a very long time.

– o O o –

Your verses do not please. The feet limp and the rhyme collapses. To make 'ocean' rhyme to 'stern' you would have to spell it 'o-shern' and that is not permissible at present, though it may be in the 'fonetik phuture'.

– o O o –

It is difficult to give you instructions in this column. You have chosen the most difficult kind of drawing - and you cannot draw. The hand should carry out the intention. It should not trust to chance; it should do exactly as it is told by the eye. Your best plan is to practice from good copies. Try such illustrations as appear in the 'B.O.P.,' the 'Century,' 'Scribner,' and the 'English Illustrated Mag-

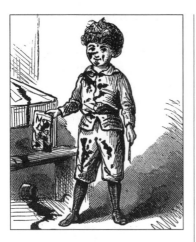

Your drawing shows no special ability, even as a copy; and your capacity for original work may be *nil.*

– o O o –

Many thanks for the offer, but the 'drawing' is scarcely up to our standard.

– o O o –

By all means join an art class ... From the specimens you send we should say that your improvement will have to be immense before you draw sufficiently well to earn a living as an artist – except on paving stones!

azine.' Begin with simple things, and endeavour to make your copy, line for line, like your original.

– o O o –

The Boy's Own Paper had a regular series of competitions where a talented few managed to get their writings, drawings, calligraphy or fretwork taken seriously. The very first competition, in 1879, was for readers to write a story based on the illustration on the next page.

The report of the results produced some interesting social insights, as well as showing how well the competitors had understood the need for an uplifting Christian tale with a moral. (At least, those were the ones that won – if there *were* any stories suggesting that the young lad was considering the house as a possible squat for him and his drug addict friends, or looking it over as a nice country pad to buy with his gambling earnings, they went ruthlessly into the waste paper basket.)

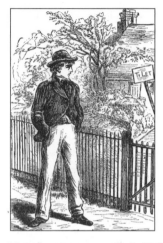

Of the stories sent in for this first competition, the majority kept pretty closely to the more obvious features of the picture. Generally, the lad was one who had disobeyed his parents and come up to London, or been self-willed and run away to sea, or had got into trouble of some kind or other, and coming home, it may be repentant, after long absence, found that while he might strive to live nobly for the future, the bygone years could neither be blotted out nor recalled. Father was, perhaps, dead, broken-hearted; and the widowed mother had had to give up her once-happy home, and find less hospitable shelter elsewhere. Well for him if he was yet in time to make some kind of amends for the past by honourable effort, and haply win back for the bereaved parent the home once her own peaceful nest. Sometimes, however, the story closes more sadly. Here is an example:–

'He had killed his mother, and the fatal words ring loudly and solemnly in his ears. Many a time he steals away, unobserved, to the quiet village churchyard, and there "beneath those rugged elms, that yew-tree's shade, Where heaves the turf in many a mould'ring heap," he weeps bitter tears of repentance over his parent's grave.'

Others, again, put the moral of their story in unmistakable language – i.e.:–

'In conclusion, we learn two great lessons from this picture: 1. That we should be obedient to our parents, and ever regard their counsel. 2. That we should scrupulously avoid evil companions and bad company.'

While yet others treat the matter quite differently, yet with very considerable skill. Thus:–

'May this short sketch induce in you a love of the beautiful, the true and the noble, and a distaste for all "harkaway" productions.' [*Jack Harkaway*' was the name of one of the more notorious 'penny dreadfuls.*]

Space will not admit of our analysing the stories in detail, but the following facts may interest many readers. Very many city boys described the 'house to let' as a fine or pretty dwelling, or even mansion; while most country lads set it down as a cottage at, say, 2s 6d a week. Numberless writers describe the lad of the picture as having been led astray by bad literature, gambling, bad companions, or drunkenness. A few give us a spoilt boy, originally with money, who gets into debt and then runs away; a still smaller number, a lad wrongly charged with theft, and so on; but as we have already said, most of the competitors kept fairly closely to their text. One of them writes in Latin.

Some of the readers competed under considerable difficulties. Or said they did, anyway. One report of a calligraphy competition quoted a letter, from a boy who had copied one of the Psalms, which an uncharitable person would suspect as an attempt to attract a sympathy vote:

I had to stand to write the Psalm. I am a cripple, and am fastened to a splint so that I can't bend my body or the injured leg. I've been five months in hospital, where I underwent four operations. I was so weak when I came out that I could hardly lift a dinner-plate off the table, and I can't sit on a chair because of the splint. When I'd written the first verse I had a good mind to give it up, my back ached so, but I managed bit by bit.

'Bravo, brave young friend!' commented the Editor, 'May the comfort and strength of the glorious words of David, upon which so many throughout the ages have drawn in moments of trial and danger, be yours to enjoy in hours of weakness and depression.'

But the boy didn't win.

One boy who did, who might well have been featured in the B.O.P. series *Some Boys Who Became Famous* (don't all famous men start as boys?) was a fifteen year old from Cheltenham, who won one guinea for a musical setting of some

> JUNIOR DIVISION (*all ages up to* 18).
>
> *Prize—One Guinea.*
>
> 4. GUSTAV VON HOLST (age 15), 1, Vittoria Walk, Cheltenham.

verses published in the previous volume. His name was Gustav von Holst. Unfortunately, the composition has not survived.

One aspect of both the competition entries and the queries that irritated the Editor was the poor standard of English displayed by some boys:

RUTHWOOD – Grammar is mental torture, is it not, particularly when you have no sense of sight or sound? 1. Does 'been' look like 'being,' or sound like it? Where are your eyes and your ears? 'Been' is past, O Ruthwood; 'being' is present. 2. And a delightful 2! 'Is it right to say them's them, or them's those?' What do they say in Darlington? 3. Charles Dickens was buried in Westminster Abbey, and the book he left unfinished was 'The Mystery of Edwin Drood.' 4. All his characters did not speak grammatically; but that was not because the author knew no better, but that he was giving the talk of ignorant persons such as you, O, Ruthwood! A phrase is not necessarily grammatical because it appears in type.

– oOo –

IGNORAMUS has as simple a way of solving his difficulty as he could wish, for 'has' is a verb, and 'as' is not.

– oOo –

We are doing our best to spread the Universal Language of the future – English, to wit – and we have something else to do than to teach Volapuk and the Panjandrum.

– oOo –

You can clean it off with turpentine or ammonia, but why 'Yours respectively'?

– oOo –

Learn to spell. When you have done so, write again. Do not trouble about boxing until you can improve on 'Proffesser'. You are not quick enough in the eyes, Wilson; you want more observing power.

– o O o –

'Chic' is not easily translatable. It is a slang expression, and you would not find it in the dictionary. It means - well, if a thing is 'chic', it is 'just the ticket', 'just the fashion', 'quite too awfully jolly' as silly people say.

– o O o –

Thanks for saying the Boy's Own Paper is a 'stunner'. We do not pretend not to know what you mean by this, nor what you mean by the word 'tin'; at the same time we must tell you that slang like this is not only vulgar, but hardly respectful.

– o O o –

Vegetable, vegetate, vegetarian. Why want to look at the dictionary at all? It is hardly worth calling such a book a dictionary if it could not give you this information.

– o O o –

TUCKERR – Decidedly no to both questions. Your letter is a caution. It contains forty-six words, and twenty of them are misspelt. Oh, Tuckerr!

AVE ATQUE VALE

LOOKING back over the *Correspondence* from the first decades of the BOY'S OWN PAPER, I find myself wondering about the reactions of at least some of the correspondents when they opened the paper some six weeks after they had written to the Editor. Surely there was some quiet blubbing by 'Milton' who, having plucked up courage to send his masterwork, a forty page poem, then read not only that it wasn't good enough for the B.O.P. but even had his fine lines about the 'circumambulatory moon' mocked in public.

Sometimes answers were given of such breathtaking callousness that it is difficult to see how the Religious Tract Society could be comfortable at their inclusion, dedicated, as it was, to Christian ideals, including, presumably, charity. In fact, there is at least one incident in the annals of the Society where the Editor was reprimanded for allowing one of Dr. Gordon Stables' answers to exceed the boundaries of good taste. To a boy who wrote, probably with great difficulty and some courage, of his 'bad habits', Stables wrote: 'Coffins are cheap and boys like you are not of much use in the world.'

At a meeting of the R.T.S. Committee, the minutes recorded that 'a grave error of judgment has been committed ... but it was in the highest interests of their correspondent.' Hutchison, as Editor, was reprimanded for allowing 'an answer which would have been improper in *any* paper' and he had to apologise on his own and Stables' behalf. The offending answer had appeared in a weekly number and the answer was changed when the issue reappeared as part of the annual volume. It now read: 'If you go on as you are, there is nothing before you but an early and dishonoured grave. Pray God to forgive and help you to resist temptation.'

Such sniping from the committee of the R.T.S went with the territory. One modern writer has said: 'The Penny Dreadfuls were not as big a threat to the BOY'S OWN PAPER as were the R.T.S. directors ...' and described the B.O.P. as 'the most important and influential juvenile periodical ever published,' a tribute to Hutchison's ability to deal diplomatically with the attempts by his own proprietors to cramp his style.

On 31 October 1899 a dinner was held in the Holborn Restaurant in London. A photograph of the assembled diners looks like any assembly of Victorian gentry. They could be Freemasons (some were) or bank employees or shareholders of a railway company. There is the usual predominance of facial hair, and a mere handful of women. Conspicuous by their absence are

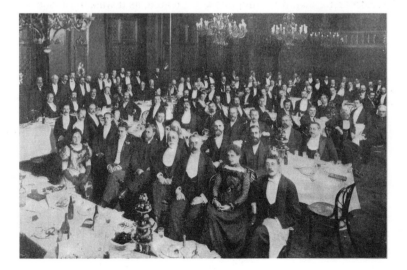

boys, which is surprising, since this dinner was, in a sense, a celebration of boyhood. It was the B.O.P 'Coming of Age' dinner, and the invited guests were the editors, writers and illustrators of the magazine, along with a selection of other guests from the higher reaches of late 19th-century English society.

The date happened to be G.A. Hutchison's birthday, and he and his wife were the guests of honour. In keeping with the spirit of much of the content of the magazine and some of its *Answers to Correspondents*, it was a very self-congratulatory affair. The dinner, described as the 'happy despatch of the appetising viands', consisted of soup, fillet of sole, whitebait, mutton cutlet, roast turkey and dessert, and then what seems to have been an endless series of toasts were drunk, interspersed with music, including a song, *The Good Old B.O.P.*, specially composed by the Rev. W.J. Foxell, M.A., B.Mus., and sung by Mr. E. Pontis Lines. 'The guests,' said a report of the dinner, 'joined in vigorously in the chorus,' which ran 'The good old "B.O.P.", the good old "B.O.P."; we know what we're about, when we raise another shout, for the good old, good old, good old "B.O.P."' There was then a presentation to Hutchison of a 'beautifully illuminated and framed address, and a cheque,' which Hutchison revealed in his speech of reply 'considerably exceeded a hundred guineas' (about £8,000 in today's purchasing power.)

The only hint in the speeches that all might not be well in the best of all nations was a reference in the toast to the Queen that 'these were troublous times, and that the Sovereign was mindful of the sufferings of her brave soldiers in South Africa.' The first phase of the Boer War had begun two weeks ago, and her brave soldiers, who no doubt included many who had sought the advice of the B.O.P. in the previous twenty-one years about how to join the services, 'had read the messages of sympathy which that womanly heart had sent out, and they would devoutly pray that the war might soon be over and that peace would be restored.' Peace was not actually restored until May 1902, by which time it had cost 75,000 lives, including 22,000 British soldiers.

When reading the account of the BOY'S OWN PAPER Coming of Age Dinner, I was reminded of another occasion where a group of individuals met in a panelled room under chandeliers and drank toasts to each other and sang songs about how splendid they all were. 'Well, I do not propose to detain you much longer,' said one speaker at this other dinner, to great applause, 'but before I resume my seat, I should like to say one word about our kind host ...' The speech on this occasion – as reported in *The Wind in the Willows* – was ironic, the 'host' was Mr Toad, whose home, Toad Hall, had been taken over by weasels. But during this dinner, Toad and Badger and Mole and Rat were gathering behind the door to the Butler's Pantry, about to burst in, reclaim Toad Hall and change the weasels' lives forever. Reading of the B.O.P. Dinner in October 1899, I could sense the 20th century waiting behind the panelling and under the flagstones and above the ceiling of the Holborn Restaurant in London.

All the certainties purveyed by 'the Editor' – embodied in Hutchison, Stables, Wood, Gordon and whoever else it was who dispensed the BOY'S OWN PAPER's bracing advice – would receive a nasty blow as the century turned and the modern age began. For a start, 'The Empire' would dwindle and there would be fewer opportunities for 'our boys' to travel out and take jobs as administrators, organising the natives and telling them what to do. 'Girls', the sisters and mothers of 'our boys', would no longer be pretty little things for whom allowances had to be made. Instead, they would fight for, and eventually get, equal voting rights, admission to universities and equal representation under the law. 'The working classes' would become 'Social classes 4 and 5' and many of them would take advantage of the increasing redistribution of wealth to become 3s, 2s or even 1s. Other races would no longer be characterised as Chinamen, niggers or kaffirs, but would gain independence in their own lands, and equal rights in ours. America and Germany, both countries presented to 'our boys' as inferior to the British race, would turn out to play parts in the 20th century world which showed where the power truly lay. And of course, those 'bad habits' that were so often coyly referred to and roundly condemned, would be replaced by a sexual revolution whose frankness and liberality

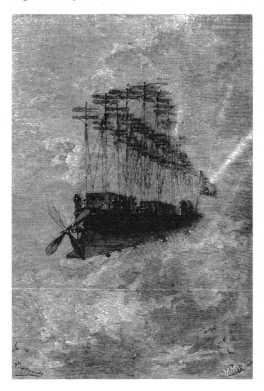

would have ignited the bushy moustaches on the faces of the middle-class, middle-aged men who tried so hard to create a race of manly boys in their own image.

But, of course, it would not all be bad. The genuine excitement that 'the Editor' shared with the boys about nature, technology, science and exploration, would increase as the 20th century saw an acceleration in the understanding of how the world works. Three months before the B.O.P. Coming of Age Dinner, two brothers, bicycle-makers in Dayton, Ohio, experimented with a way of adjusting the shape of a man-made wing which led, in 1903, to powered flight. By a hundred years after the B.O.P. Dinner, people-carriers were flying in the sky that would have been beyond even the wildest imagination of that very successful serial writer, M. Jules Verne.

Darwin's ideas on evolution by natural selection transformed ideas about the biological world in a way which, however much the B.O.P. admired Darwin's 'shrewd powers of observation and patient industry', would have shocked its evangelical Christian founders. Perhaps it was a relief that the Rev. J.G. Wood, recipient of so many crushed beetles, desiccated caterpillars and putrefied squirrels in the post, had died before the end of the century.

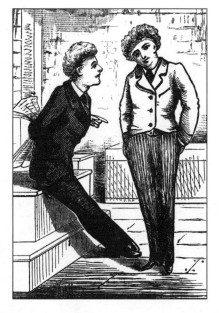

The BOY'S OWN PAPER was actually to see and report on many of these developments before it finally closed down in 1967, but that was in the hands of a new generation of Editors who treated 'their boys' more gently. Fewer and fewer boys were told things like 'You are killing yourself', 'When we are extremely hard up for new ideas we will avail ourselves of your suggestion', 'You have evidently mistaken your gifts', 'Be content with the mischief you have done, and do it no more', or 'You cruel boy'.

Where the 19th century saw boys, and some men, treated as 'our boys', which meant that they were assumed to be manly, white, British and Christian, the 20th century was eventually to see the idea spread that everyone – boys, girls, men and women, white, black and yellow – should be treated as people. And it was to be a century when the idea grew that people could be helped rather than condemned, and that nobody deserved to be told that 'your case is hopeless'.